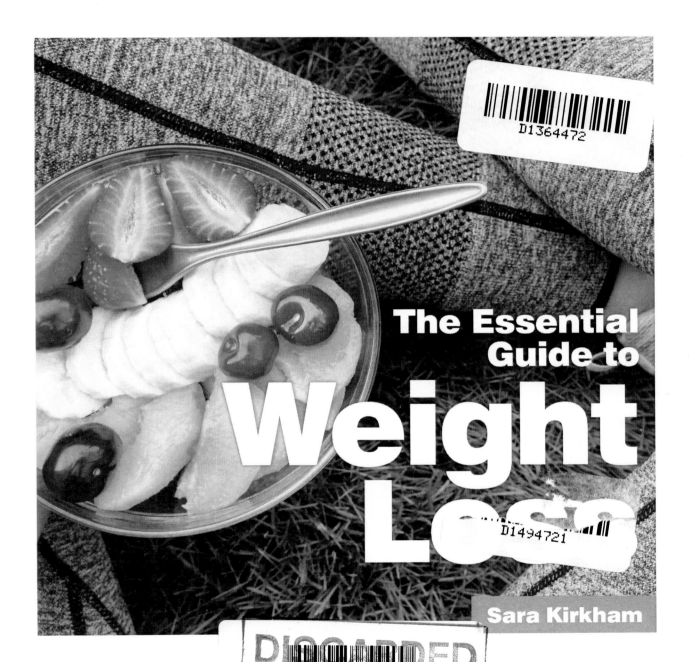

The Essential Guide to
Weight Loss

Sara Kirkham

Published in Great Britain in 2018 by
need2know
Remus House
Coltsfoot Drive
Peterborough
PE2 9BF
Telephone 01733 898103
www.need2knowbooks.co.uk

Contents

Introduction

I n a world saturated with dietary advice, this book is a source of credible information and metabolic insights, with indispensable, practical weight loss tips, providing all the tools you will need to achieve long term successful weight loss. You'll find a critical review of today's most popular diets too, helping you to choose the right 'diet' for you.

It has been estimated that almost 50% of women are dieting most of the time, with over 13 million people on a permanent diet. Yet despite these figures, we aren't getting any slimmer – obesity is a disease epidemic. The vast majority of people with a chronic weight problem have inflammatory and metabolic issues caused by elevated insulin levels – the cause, effects and remedy to this are discussed within this book. Many people following a weight loss regime will falter within the first few weeks, re-gain any weight lost, and resume with an alternative diet plan, only to fail again. This book is for every person still looking for the ultimate guide that will enable them to lose weight and maintain it, whilst eating a healthy, balanced diet.

Although the basic principle behind weight loss is simple (if you take in fewer calories than you use up, you will lose weight), weight loss is certainly not easy to achieve for many people. There are countless factors and pressures that contribute to our food choices, and making dietary or lifestyle changes is inherently difficult. We tend to set goals that are too ambitious, follow diets that cannot be maintained, and quickly become disillusioned with the results. This book will enable you to understand weight gain and weight loss – it explains how your metabolic rate affects the amount of calories you need, and discusses the most effective ways to lose weight. It will enable you to take stock of where you are, and set realistic diet and exercise goals to achieve success.

Weight Loss – The Essential Guide is the ultimate guide to weight loss If you want to...

- Finally succeed with successfully losing weight and keeping it off
- Learn how to set realistic weight loss goals that are more likely to be successful
- Discover how to improve your metabolism to succeed with long term weight loss
- Reduce calorie intake and/or increase metabolism without being 'on a diet'
- Discover the best way to lose weight – is it fasting, paleo, keto, low carb or low fat?

- Understand how to control your appetite, blood sugar levels and eating behaviours, and get back in control of what you eat
- Understand the psychology behind changing your eating behaviour
- Discover how to have a long-term exercise regime to promote weight loss.

Disclaimer

This book is not intended to replace professional medical advice, although it can be used alongside the advice of your doctor. If you are considering making dietary or lifestyle changes, you are recommended to consult a qualified professional such as a nutritionist or dietician, and if you have any health issues, or are obese, it is recommended that you consult a healthcare professional.

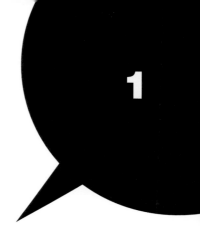

1

Globesity – The New Epidemic

Weight loss is big business. 26% of adults in the UK are classed as obese, compared with 7% in 1980 (NHS, 2017). Over 650 million people around the world are obese, and 52% of adults are overweight or obese (World Health Organisation, 2016) – worldwide obesity levels almost tripled between 1975 and 2016, and show few signs of reducing. Whilst some experts suggest that the obesity epidemic is caused by an increased intake of energy-dense foods that are high in fat and sugars, together with a reduction in physical activity, more recent research has indicated that dietary guidelines over the last two to three decades recommending high-carbohydrate, low-fat diets as the universal panacea are deeply flawed. Obesity has increased since the availability of low fat foods and diets higher in sugar and starches have grown, emboldened by slimming clubs and even health promotion organisations.

A growing problem

It's a simple equation: if energy in is greater than energy out, we gain weight. However, weight loss may be simple in theory, but it is not necessarily easy in practice. Changing our eating and lifestyle habits is often difficult to do, and is not always helped by the plethora of weight loss and dieting information available with constant high profile marketing... magazines, diet books, celebrity diets, television programmes and the internet all provide a vast and constantly changing source of information about how to lose weight – but which sources can you trust?

The promise of quick results entices us to follow harsh and unhealthy diets that may initially create weight loss (though not necessarily loss of body fat), but are not sustainable for any length of time. So you return to your normal eating pattern and regain any lost weight. Then you look for the next diet to try.

Why do we get fat?

Body fat accumulates when we take in more calories than we use up. It's a simple equation known as the Energy Balance Equation: for weight maintenance, calories in must equal calories out. However, calculating our calorie consumption and expenditure is difficult and often inaccurate, so achieving an energy balance can be challenging.

Having such a wide range of taste-enhanced, cheap food available is too much of a temptation for many of us, and when coupled with food marketing gimmicks such as 'two for one', tasty snacks placed at crucial locations in supermarkets to tempt us, even smells piped into supermarkets to stimulate the first stage of digestion and entice us into buying fresh bread and bakery products – how can we resist?

On top of this, our lives revolve around food... we have recognized meal times whether we are hungry or not, business lunches and sandwich runs in the office, and events throughout the year where indulgence is not only accepted but expected, such as Christmas, Easter, holidays or birthdays.

If you have ever dieted before, you will know that there is always something round the corner that gets in the way of your diet or healthy eating plan. Many people do not eat to live, but live to eat! Food is no longer just an energy source: we use food for comfort and for social acceptance, we eat and drink to celebrate and commiserate, and we even eat to congratulate or punish our dieting achievements and downfalls.

How do we get fat?

After a meal, a hormone called insulin tells our cells to absorb glucose, and increases the uptake of triglycerides and some amino acids. Insulin stimulates the body to build glycogen from glucose, make proteins from amino acids, and store more fat.

When excess food energy is consumed, anything that cannot be used for energy or for other purposes in the body (such as building hormones and cell walls for example) can be converted into body fat (adipose tissue) and stored. We can convert excess carbohydrates, proteins or fats into adipose tissue, although it takes more energy to convert carbohydrates and proteins into body fat. For example, 100 excess fat calories can be stored using approximately 2 – 3 calories of energy, but 100 excess calories of glucose (carbohydrate) will take about 23 calories to convert it into fat and store it.

We only store approximately 2000 calories of glucose as stored carbohydrate energy (glycogen), and once these stores are full in the liver and muscles, excess glucose not used for energy will be converted into adipose tissue. Excess protein can also be converted into fat and stored. Fat (and excess glucose or protein converted into fat) is stored in fat cells called adipocytes. Although increased dietary intake and body fat levels during childhood and adolescence multiply the number of fat cells we develop, once past this growth phase, the number of fat cells we have generally remains the same unless we overeat. Adipocytes grow in size as they store more fat and the fat droplet inside expands, and reduce in size as fat is used up for energy and weight is lost. Weight regain can involve both hypertrophy (growth of adipose cells) and hyperplasia (multiplication of fat cells).

'It doesn't matter how many fat cells you have, but how much fat you put inside them.'

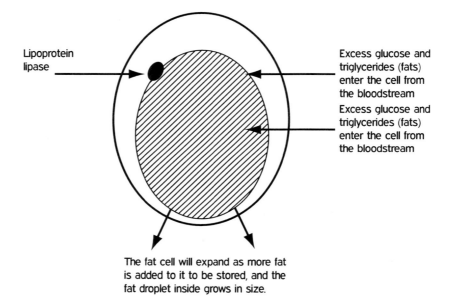

An adipocyte containing a fat droplet

Lipoprotein lipase

Excess glucose and triglycerides (fats) enter the cell from the bloodstream

Excess glucose and triglycerides (fats) enter the cell from the bloodstream

The fat cell will expand as more fat is added to it to be stored, and the fat droplet inside grows in size.

'We are more likely to form a greater number of fat cells during the first few years of life, and between age nine to 13.'

We can store a lot of energy as fat because it is stored without water, so it is relatively lightweight and compact. One pound of adipose tissue contains approximately 3500 calories, so to remove this amount of fat from the body we have to create an energy deficit of slightly less than 3500 calories, either by eating less or exercising more. It is slightly less as we use some of this energy up just converting the stored fat back into triglycerides to break it down for energy.

Human behavior causes obesity

If you live in an environment that has caused obesity in others, there is an increased chance that you will also gain excess weight. Some research has shown that people who are overweight are more likely to have overweight pets because they are more likely to over feed them, as they do themselves. The human behaviour experienced in our formative years also contributes to our lifetime eating habits.

Think back to your childhood...

- Were food portions large?

- Were you encouraged to finish your plate, regardless of how full you felt?

- Did you have to finish your main meal before you could have a dessert?

- Were all meals finished with something sweet?

- Were sweets and confectionary used as treats?

- Were meals rushed or eaten on the go, encouraging you to eat quickly?

All of these behaviours contribute to poor eating habits, encouraging over eating, eating too quickly to recognize and respond to satiety (feeling full), or creating a sweet tooth in later years. We tend to continue with known and preferred eating habits until there is either a deliberate or life-changing occurrence in our life. This can be a decision to change eating habits for weight loss or health reasons, but is just as likely to be a change in job, moving home to live with a new partner or different family member, going to university or living abroad.

What do I have to gain by losing weight?

Several health conditions are caused or exaggerated by excess body fat levels, including Type 2 diabetes, insulin resistance and metabolic syndrome, coronary heart disease, osteoarthritis, liver diseases and some types of cancer. Adipose tissue, particularly if stored around the middle, also releases inflammatory substances into the body that can cause further health complications. As fat cells grow larger, they secrete a protein that reduces fat cell metabolism, so we use up less fat.

In addition to the physical stresses on the body, our body shape affects the way we feel about ourselves, and causes a range of behavioural problems ranging from low self esteem and poor self confidence to depression. It can affect the way that we dress and present ourselves to others, and often influences the decisions we make in life, such as whether we feel comfortable going to a fitness class or swimming, or whether we apply for a promotion at work. It also has an effect upon our relationships with other people.

'Losing 10kg can reduce blood pressure by 10mmHg, reduce total cholesterol by 10%, LDL cholesterol by 15%, triglycerides by 30% and fasting blood glucose by 50%. HDL 'good' cholesterol can be increased by 8%.'

Lose weight – live longer

Being a healthy weight also appears to be linked with longevity. Animal research has shown that calorie restriction can extend life expectancy by one third to twice as long as normal and this is also illustrated in a number of human populations.

Benefits of losing weight

- Reduced risk of disease
- Increased longevity
- Improved quality of life
- Higher self esteem and improved self confidence
- Better body image
- Easier to get around.

'In some areas of Japan where up to 40% fewer calories are consumed than in other areas, there are more centenarians and much less disease.'

Weigh it up

But even once you have acknowledged all the benefits of weight loss, there is still one big hurdle – you will have to make substantial changes to your eating habits and lifestyle in order to be successful – and this is where the sticking point is for most people. Making changes like this can be tough, and requires will power and support as well as know how and motivation. That is where this book can help, because here you will find not only a trustworthy source of information, but also an insight into how you can change your eating behaviours for life – and stick with it.

Summing Up

- We gain weight when we take in more calories than we use up

- Many people live to eat rather than eat to live

- Any type of excess food can be converted into body fat and stored

- We form more fat cells during early life and adolescent growth phases

- When we consume more carbohydrate, protein or fat than the body needs, all these nutrients are converted into fat and stored in adipocytes

- Adipocytes initially fill up as more fat is stored, but we can develop a greater number of fat cells too

- Once you have developed additional fat cells, you are stuck with them, but it is the amount of fat you store within these cells that determines your body fat level

- Being overweight contributes to a number of other disease conditions.

2

How Do You Measure Up?

There are several ways to measure your weight or the amount of body fat you are carrying – each measuring option has its own benefits and drawbacks, so just choose a way to measure your weight loss that suits you – as long as the results are going in the right direction, it doesn't matter if you measure overall body weight on the scales, girth measurements with a tape measure, or body fat percentage. However, waist measurements and body fat percentage are more accurate measures of body fat and its associated health risks than overall weight or BMI.

Body Mass Index

Body Mass Index is based upon height and weight, and provides a figure that places you on a chart such as the one below. However, research has found that some people with a normal BMI but a large waist/hip ratio have increased risk of death during follow-up compared to people with a smaller waist/hip ratio, illustrating that if you carry weight around the middle but are otherwise quite slim, the BMI may look favourable, but this is not an accurate way to predict health risks or even find out if you are 'over fat' as opposed to being overweight. However, this is the measurement your doctor is currently likely to use to assess whether you are a healthy weight or not.

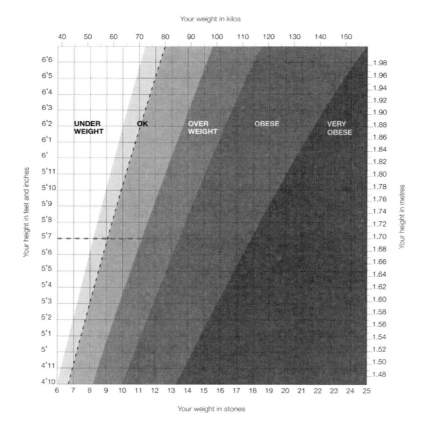

© Crown copyright. Source: Food Standards Agency.

It is also important to remember that this measurement does not take into account the amount of muscle (lean tissue) that you have. For example, if you exercise regularly, the extra muscle will increase your weight, yet you may carry less body fat than someone of the same weight as you. If your BMI seems unduly high, it may be worth having your body fat levels checked with a health and fitness professional, or checking your waist circumference or waist/hip ratio.

Calculating your Body Mass Index

1 Convert your weight into kilograms (if your scales show your weight in kilograms, skip to number 2).

First of all, write down your weight in pounds. For example, if you weigh 10 stones 8 lbs, multiply 10 by 14 (because there are 14 pounds in each stone), and then add on the 8lbs to give your total weight in pounds. In this example it would be as follows:

10 x 14 = 140 + 8 = 148lbs

Now convert this into kilograms by dividing it by 2.2.

For example… 148 divided by 2.2 = 67.27kg

2 Convert your height into metres.

You can either use a conversion chart for this, or convert feet and inches into metres as follows. (If you know your height in metres, skip to the next part where we calculate your height^2).

3 Write down your height in inches. For example, if you are 5 feet 5 inches tall, multiply 5 by 12 (because there are 12 inches in each foot), and then add on the extra 5 inches to give your total height in inches. In this example it would be as follows:

5 x 12 = 60 + 5 = 65 inches

Now convert this into centimeters by multiplying it by 2.54.

For example… 65 multiplied by 2.54 = 165.1cm

And now divide this by 100 to convert it into metres…

165.1cm divided by 100 = 1.65 metres.

Before you can calculate your Body Mass Index, you need to do a further calculation by multiplying your height in metres by the same figure again. This gives you your height^2 (squared).

Using our example of a height of 1.65 metres…

$1.65 \times 1.65 = 2.72m^2$.

Now you have your weight in kg and your height in metres^2, you can calculate your Body Mass Index.

3) Body Mass Index (BMI) = weight (kg) divided by height (m^2).

Now divide your weight (in kg) by your height (in m^2) to give you your BMI. In this example, the Body Mass Index is calculated as follows:

67.27kg divided by 2.72m = 24.73.

Now check out your Body Mass Index (BMI) below.

- BMI of 18-24.9 is desirable
- BMI of 25-30 is considered overweight
- BMI of 30+ is considered obese
- BMI of 40+ is considered morbidly obese

You can also input your weight and height into calculators on various websites and let them work it out for you! Try this one on the NHS website at **https://www.nhs.uk/Tools/ Pages/Healthyweightcalculator.aspx**.

Tape measurements

This sounds really simple, and it is one of the quickest and easiest ways to monitor your progress as you lose weight. However, it can be inaccurate if not done carefully, lifting spirits one month only to drop you into despair when you appear to have gained back the inches you thought you had already lost.

Considerations for an accurate measurement

1 Take measurements on bare skin – clothes make measurements inaccurate and can easily add centimeters to a measurement – and you won't remember what you wore in your last measure up!

2 Note the exact spot that you are measuring – use clear 'body landmarks' to line up your tape measure, such as the bellybutton for a waist measurement, or the hip bones for a hip measurement. For arm and leg measurements you can measure how many inches/centimeters from the crotch or elbow your measuring point is, or use birthmarks/tattoos to help line up your tape measure. Write down exactly where you measured so you can repeat the measurement in the same place.

3 Take up any slack in the tape measure and make sure it isn't twisted.

4 Have someone else take the measurements – as well as this being much more accurate, they are more likely to be objective (and not pull the tape measure in tighter on subsequent measurements!).

5 Take the measurement without looking at the previous figure – seeing what you were last week/last month may lead you to inadvertently move the tape measure around until you find a measurement that is slightly less than the previous figure.

6 Don't attempt to hold in your stomach – you're only cheating yourself!

7 Take the measurements at the same time of day if possible, avoiding obvious things that could affect a net change in girth measurements such as measuring immediately after eating.

8 Keep a clear record of your measurements in a diary, on a calendar, or on a sheet of paper kept in a safe place – figures jotted down on a scrap of paper are too easily lost and you will not remember measurements from a month ago.

Remember, as you lose body fat from all over the body, you will lose different amounts from different areas. Doing girth measurements will give you an idea of where you are losing the most weight from (if you haven't already figured this out from the way your clothes are fitting). Contrary to popular belief, you cannot spot reduce body fat from specific areas, although you can tone up the muscle in targeted parts of the body.

Waist circumference

Adipose tissue held around the thighs and bottom is not as much of a health risk as excess fat stored around the middle. Central obesity increases the lipid (fat) levels in the liver's blood supply, decreasing the liver's sensitivity to insulin (a hormone that reduces blood glucose levels) and contributing to the development of Type 2 diabetes. The elevated blood lipids from stored adipose tissue around the middle also increase the production of low density lipoprotein cholesterol ('bad' cholesterol) in the liver, which can contribute to cardiovascular disease if it becomes oxidized. So, it is a good idea to keep your waist circumference within specific circumference guidelines, and this provides an easy-to-measure goal for weight loss and improved health.

Knowing your waist circumference or waist-hip ratio can help you to discover whether you are storing excess calories around the middle, and also give you an easy way to measure your weight loss – with a tape measure! Here are the recommended guidelines suggested by the NHS.

'The 'apple' shape is less desirable than the 'pear' shape as far as health goes: adipose tissue around the abdomen is linked with increased risk of Type 2 diabetes, coronary heart disease and inflammatory endocrine disorders.'

Waist circumference guidelines for women	Waist circumference guidelines for men
Ideal: less than 80cm (32 inches) High: 80cm to 88cm (32 to 35 inches) Very high: more than 88cm (35 inches)	Ideal: less than 94cm (37 inches) High: 94cm to 102cm (37 to 40 inches) Very high: more than 102cm (40 inches)

(NHS, 2018).

For people of South Asian origin there is an even greater health risk linked with central obesity, with waist measurements of 80cm in women and 90cm in men putting health at risk. Due to the rise in obesity and therefore a general shift in population 'norms', several organisations indicate that waist circumferences of over 88cm for women and over 102cm for men present a significantly increased risk of Type 2 diabetes and cardiovascular disease.

How to measure your waist circumference

Locate the top of your hip bone on one side of the body, and then locate the bottom of your ribs on the same side. Halfway between the two bones is your waist – this will usually be at around the same level as your bellybutton, and at the narrowest part of your torso. You may find it easier to do this (and to see the tape measurement) using a mirror. The Ashwell Shape Chart © below illustrates how your waist measurement might be affecting your health: this could be used as an additional motivational tool as you lose weight and move from one section of the chart to another.

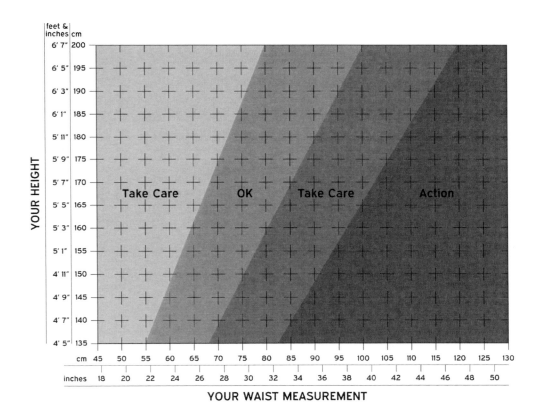

'Increased mortality risk related to excess body fat is mainly due to abdominal adiposity.'
Bigaard et al, 2005.

© Crown copyright. Source: Food Standards Agency.

Waist-hip ratio

Your waist-hip ratio compares the circumference of your waist to your hips – the greater your waist circumference is in comparison to your hips (the more 'apple' shaped you are), the higher the level of central obesity and health risks.

Waist-hip ratios

Women	Men
Ideal: less than 0.8 Too high: 0.85 or more	Ideal: less than 0.90 Too high: 1 or more

How to calculate your waist-hip ratio

To calculate your waist-hip ratio, simply divide your waist measurement by your hip measurement. For example, if your waist measurement was 80cm and your hips measured 110cm, your waist-hip ratio would be 0.72.

$$\frac{\text{Waist } 80}{\text{Hips } 110} = 0.72$$

Make sure that both measurements are either in inches or in centimeters.

'A high waist-to-hip ratio is directly linked with increased risk of coronary heart disease.'

Using scales

Probably the most widely used and convenient device for measuring weight loss is weighing scales. However, when you step onto a set of scales you are weighing everything – lean tissue, bone mass, stored glycogen (carbohydrate energy), water and adipose (fat) tissue – so if you are quite muscular, your weight in comparison to someone else can appear quite heavy, yet you may not be overweight. Lean tissue (muscle) is much heavier than fatty tissue, so the more muscle you have, the heavier you will be. Conversely, fatty tissue is stored without added water and doesn't weigh as much for the same volume, one reason why weight (fat) loss on the scales can seem so slow. As with other forms of measurement, scales can also be inaccurate, so take these tips into account for a fair measure...

- For scales with a needle gauge, always make sure the pointer is set to zero before you get on.

- If you can't see where the needle is from where you are standing, have someone else take the reading. This will be more accurate anyway, as the angle at which you look at the needle can affect your reading.

need2know

- For electronic scales, if the measurement seems to fluctuate or is much more or less than expected, check the battery.

- Always stand upright – leaning forwards or backwards can affect the result.

- Weigh yourself naked if possible to omit any weight changes due to heavy clothes or shoes. If not possible to weigh yourself naked, at least remove shoes and heavy items of clothing.

- Stand weighing scales on a solid floor surface such as wood or stone rather than carpet, and always weigh yourself on the same scales, and the same floor surface.

What should my weight be?

You can use the weight/height chart shown earlier on as a guide, but remember that different body types will affect what a normal weight should be. There are three general somatotypes, or body shapes:

- Ectomorphs which are slender, small boned, and generally carry little body fat with a low body weight

- Mesomorphs which have a muscular build and therefore have a body weight that can be high in proportion to body fat levels

- Endomorphs which tend to carry higher levels of body fat and have a more rounded body shape.

The more lean tissue (muscle) you have, the heavier you will weigh on the scales. Due to this anomaly, you may want to use an additional form of measurement to assess changes in body shape, such as tape measurements.

Body fat measuring devices

There are several devices that measure body fat levels – most of the home measurement devices use something called impedance. A very light electrical current is sent around the body, usually from one foot to the other, or from fingertips to toes, and the speed of the current is measured. An electrical current travels at different speeds through fatty tissue, muscle, bone and water, and so estimations about the proportion of water, lean and fatty tissue are made and displayed on the measuring device. The actual weights of water, muscle and fat given are based upon the proportions of each type of tissue from the impedance results, so your hydration level (the amount of water in the body) can affect the results significantly, and it is recommended that you maintain adequate hydration for each measurement – obviously accurate changes in body fat levels can only be gathered if hydration levels are kept fairly constant. Some scales have in-built impedance, enabling you to measure total body weight, lean mass (muscle) and body fat levels, and other devices (BodyStat, Omron) measure impedance through the body without total body weight (which is entered separately).

The benefits of measuring body fat are:

- As you only want to lose adipose tissue (fat) and no lean tissue, this allows you to monitor the type of tissue you are losing

- When overall weight loss is slow this can be very frustrating – knowing that lean tissue weight has increased but body fat levels have dropped is very motivating, as this will increase metabolism and assist further fat loss.

Many 'fad' diets result in weight loss through reductions in water or muscle weight, or reduced stores of carbohydrate (glycogen). This may look good on the scales, but does not show a reduction in body fat (which is the type of tissue you want to lose), and the weight is often regained very easily as soon as fluids or carbohydrates are taken in. Measuring and monitoring body fat levels can help you to lose weight more gradually and prevent drastic reductions in water, glycogen and lean tissue, which are all counterproductive to a long term reduction in adipose tissue and maintained weight loss.

How to measure your weight loss

- Body Mass Index (BMI)

- Tape measurements – choose from waist circumference, waist-hip ratio, or a selection of girth measurements taken from the areas you want to reduce (waist, stomach, hips, thighs, arms etc.)

- Scales

- Device measuring body fat percentage

Benefits and drawbacks of measuring instruments

Type of measurement	✓	✗
Tape measurements	Quick and easy Waist and waist/hip ratio are linked to health risks too	Can be inaccurate
Scales	Quick and easy Accurate measure of overall weight loss (dependent upon scales used)	Measure total body weight so it is unknown what type of weight (water weight, body fat or lean tissue) has been lost
Body Mass Index (BMI)	Easy with web-based BMI calculators	Only based upon weight and height – it can provide an 'overweight' reading for heavy-muscled individuals and is not an accurate predictor of health. BMI changes slowly so can be a little demotivating
Body fat measurements	Measures changes in body fat, which is the type of tissue you ideally want to lose	Measures are affected by hydration levels, which can be difficult to keep the same to monitor accurate changes

Summing Up

- Choose a type of measurement that you have easy access to

- Make sure your measurements are accurate

- Write your measurements down

- Don't forget to put the date each measurement was taken

- Decide how often you are going to take each measurement

- Choosing more than one type of measurement can reveal a more accurate picture of changes in body shape, and can also provide ongoing motivation when one measurement appears to show no or little change, but another measurement shows clear progress.

So now you have an idea of how you measure up, but before you start on your weight loss regime, let's find out what a successful weight loss goal looks like.

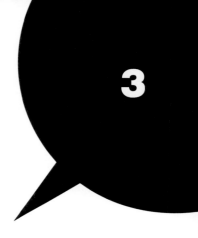

3

Planning for Success

The biggest question on everyone's lips is how to lose weight and keep it off, but with the plethora of diets and weight loss solutions bombarding us from every angle, it's not always easy to know what to do. However, with the right dietary advice and a sensible long term plan, you can follow a healthy, sustainable diet, balance calorie intake and expenditure, and enjoy successful, life-long weight maintenance.

Reasons for weight gain

There are three key reasons why we gain weight:

- We eat too many high calorie foods or foods with hidden calories
- Our portion sizes are too large – we may be eating the right foods but are simply eating too much of them

- We aren't active enough to use up the calories we have consumed. This is common when a change in job or lifestyle has resulted in lower activity levels, but we haven't adjusted our diet to reduce calorie intake accordingly.

Other chapters in this book discuss how various diets may create weight loss, and whilst all calories were not quite created equal (see Chapter 5), and different ways of eating may create metabolic changes in the body that favour weight loss (Chapter 8), a calorie deficit does have to be created in order to lose weight.

Before we look at how you're going to reduce your calorie intake, or increase your energy expenditure, you need to set your first weight loss goal. Once you know how much weight you plan to lose, you'll also know what sort of calorie deficit you have to achieve, and this will indicate how many changes need to be made to your usual daily food intake.

How much weight should you lose?

A reasonable guideline for your first weight loss goal is to lose 5% of your body weight over six weeks. If you have a BMI or waist measurement that places you as obese, you may be able to safely lose 10% of your body weight over this time period. This is easy to calculate as follows.

Calculating how much weight to lose

To calculate 5% of your body weight, multiply your weight in pounds (or kg) by 5, then divide by 100. Using the earlier example of a body weight of 148 lbs, this gives us…

148 x 5 = 740, divided by 100 = 7.4lbs

In this example, 7.4lbs is 5% of total body weight, and provides the first weight loss goal. To lose this weight over a six week period, you would need to lose 1.2lbs weekly (just divide the weight loss goal you have by 6 as follows):

7.4lbs divided by 6 weeks = 1.2lbs weight loss weekly.

Six weeks is a good time period to use when setting short term goals. Remember, this is just your first small weight loss goal, and does not necessarily represent the total amount of weight you might want to lose.

If 5% of your current weight divided over 6 weeks comes to more than 2lbs weekly weight loss, it's worth planning the weight loss over 8 weeks, or simply limiting your weekly weight loss to 2lb, to make sure it's realistic. This is because many weight loss goals fail if they are based upon an unachievable weekly weight loss. Don't worry if you would like to lose more weight than this – the goal is not a limit, and any weight lost in addition to the original goal set is a bonus! Here are some helpful guidelines to help you set and achieve your first weight loss goal.

Setting successful weight loss goals

The way to successful weight loss that is sustainable is through making small changes and taking small steps. This way, your lifestyle is less disrupted and you can continue successfully. Once the new changes become a habit, you can make further changes. It is a common mistake to aim for the total weight loss you want (e.g. 2 stone) without breaking it down into smaller goals.

Deciding on your initial weight loss goal

Many people think that losing 1 – 2lbs a week is insignificant. However, when you consider how much of a calorie loss you would have to achieve in order to lose two pounds a week, you may reconsider. There are approximately 3,500 calories in 1lb of fat, so to lose 2lb of fat a week, you have to create a calorie deficit of approximately 7000 calories over the week, or eat 1000 calories less a day! This is a tall order for most people, and is unrealistic unless you have a lot of weight to lose, or are currently consuming a very high calorie diet. Even losing 1lb weekly requires a calorie deficit of 3,500 calories a week, or 500 calories daily.

It's also worth considering that the less weight you have to lose, the less body fat you are likely to lose each week. So if you have a stone or less to lose, aim for a smaller loss such as half a pound weekly. It's better to achieve the goal you originally set, rather than begin with an unrealistic target and then fail. A loss of half a pound weekly would still create an overall weight loss of nearly half a stone over 12 weeks. In Chapter 4 we'll look at your food diary to see where you might find calories to cut out, but for now, let's agree on your weight loss goal.

'Smart goals can increase your chance of success by up to 20%.'

SMART goals

Setting SMART goals for weight loss will increase your chances of success. SMART stands for goals that are…

S pecific
M easurable
A chievable
R ealistic
T ime-bound

Setting your SMART weight loss goal

1 Choose a specific goal, such as the weight you want to be at the end of 6 weeks, a specific lower waist measurement, or a reduced body fat percentage.

2 Make sure it's measurable, and take account of the guidelines for each form of measurement to ensure accurate results. Your measure could be your weight on the scales, a tape measurement or your waist-hip ratio.

3 Make sure your goal is achievable and realistic – although you will naturally want weight loss results as quickly as possible, setting yourself a tough goal is likely to end in failure, which is de-motivating and often contributes to comfort eating and further weight gain.

4 Your goal must have an end date when you will achieve it by. Decide on a date by which you will achieve your first weight loss goal – if you have an important event that you would like to lose weight for, such as a wedding, holiday or social occasion, you might want to use this date as your goal if it's within 4 to 8 weeks.

How do I know if my weight loss goal is realistic?

Gauging whether your weight loss goal is realistic to achieve can be difficult at first. As a general guideline, if your Body Mass Index, body fat or tape measurement placed you in the 'very obese' category, you may be able to lose 2lbs or more weekly – the more weight you have to lose, the easier it is to lose more weight each week. If you are obese, you may be able to lose half a pound to a pound weekly, and if you are overweight, just aim for half a pound a week. Calculating 5% of your current body weight and using that as an initial weight loss guideline is a good place to start, but if you have been trying to lose weight unsuccessfully, or weight loss has recently stalled, you may need to set

'Six weeks is thought to be the best period of time for successful goal setting – it's not too far away that you delay your weight loss action, and it is close enough to keep you motivated.'

a smaller weight loss goal. As you lose weight, you will become more adept at setting yourself realistic goals as you get to know your body, and be able to judge how much weight you can expect to lose.

Take these things into consideration:

- How much you currently weigh and how much weight you have to lose
- Whether you have already lost weight and at what rate are you currently losing weight each week
- Whether your weight loss has slowed down or hit a plateau
- How much exercise you will be able to do
- How much you are willing to change your diet
- Whether there is anything that might get in the way of your weight loss goal, such as social occasions or holidays.

It is important to be realistic and not set an unachievable goal – this is a common error, as we let our hopes override common sense. However, even if you are losing weight, you may lose motivation if you realise you are not going to achieve the weight loss goal you have set for yourself, and this can be detrimental to your success.

For example, if you set a weight loss goal to lose one stone over six weeks and lost 12lbs you may feel disappointed because you didn't hit your weight loss target. However, if you set a weight loss goal of 10lbs over six weeks and lost 12lbs, you will feel motivated as you over-achieved your target. The weight lost is the same in both examples, but the level of motivation and feeling of achievement is different, and may affect whether you continue with your weight loss efforts or not. The idea is not to set a goal that is easy to achieve, but to decide upon an achievable, realistic weight loss goal.

'You are not limited by a realistic weight loss goal – if you lose more weight than you originally planned, this will motivate you even more!'

Write it down and tell others

It's important to write your plans down so that you know what your measurements and goals are, and when you will be measuring your success. Write it in your diary, mark it on the calendar, maybe even plan to treat yourself (not with chocolates!) when you reach your first goal weight. Telling others of your goal may also help you to succeed, as once you have verbalised what you intend to achieve, you are more likely to set out to succeed and meet other people's expectations as well as your own.

Process and outcome goals

The usual way to measure weight loss is with a weight, body fat or tape measurement – these are all known as outcome goals as they measure the end result rather than the process of the goal (what you are doing to achieve the outcome goal). Research into the success of goal setting has shown that outcome based goals are likely to be less successful than process-orientated goals for the following reasons:

The outcome (end result) of a weight loss plan is not entirely in your control, it is only as a result of the process

You have to wait a period of time to measure the outcome, and many of us need ongoing motivation to keep us going.

'Measure the journey, not the destination.'

You have more control over process goals; for example, you can determine how many exercise minutes you complete in a week, but you can't determine exactly how much weight you will lose. If you enjoy the daily/weekly success of achieving what you need to do to lose weight (e.g. exercising or sticking to specific dietary changes), this is likely to keep you motivated to stick with your new regime, as well as confirm that you are on track for success. Naturally, you can simply weigh or measure yourself each week, but these measurements are likely to be unpredictable (weight) and slow to change (body fat and tape measurements).

Of course you can set yourself both an outcome goal, such as a target weight to get to, and a process goal that determines how you are going to achieve the weight loss. Here are some examples of process goals:

- Complete 180 minutes of exercise each week
- Limit alcohol units to 14 units per week
- Swap your usual breakfast to fruit salad every day
- Reduce a breakfast cereal portion size to 30g.

You can also set more than one process goal to help you achieve your outcome (but limit yourself to a maximum of three goals to keep it simple). If you have struggled with achieving weight loss in the past, setting process goals and focusing on the journey rather than the destination could be the key to your success.

Summing Up

So, armed with the following information from this chapter you are ready to begin your weight loss plan. You know...

- How much weight you should aim to lose for your first weight loss target, and
- How to set a successful weight loss goal.

Remember, your weight loss goal should be SMART for success:

1 Set a specific goal to achieve

2 Decide how you will measure your progress (weight, tape measurements, exercise minutes etc.)

3 Make sure it's achievable and realistic

4 Note down the date that you aim to achieve it by – ideally four to six weeks time.

Now let's take a look at how you're going to do it!

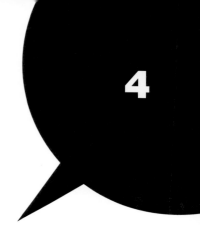

4

How to Create a Calorie Deficit with Diet

There are three ways to create a calorie deficit:

- Reducing your calorie intake
- Using up more calories through activity and exercise
- Eating less and exercising more.

Reducing your calorie intake

Rather than randomly cutting foods out of your diet (as in many fad diets), for long term success it's worth taking a more considered approach. If you cut out all the foods you enjoy eating, your weight loss will be short lived, and any long term eating habit must be nutritionally sound and healthy. Adjusting your current diet to one that is healthier and contains fewer calories can be much easier than trying to follow a completely different eating regime. In theory, if you simply make a few changes that reduce your energy intake, you will lose weight. If you choose to change poor eating habits that are daily or very regular, you may lose all the weight you want or need to, without having to 'go on a diet'.

The first thing to think about is whether you eat a lot of foods that are high in calories. These are foods such as fatty meats, spreads, dips and oils, alcohol, cakes, biscuits and confectionary. You can check the calorie content of foods at **www.weightlossresources. co.uk** or on a calorie/fitness tracker such as My Fitness Pal. However, knowing which foods to avoid and actually reducing these foods are two different things! One of the best ways to help you cut calories from your diet is by keeping a written or online food diary. Once you have noted everything that you eat and drink, this helps you to spot where excess calories are being consumed, and you can plan how to reduce your daily calorie intake.

Using a food diary

Food diaries or calorie trackers have to be completed every day, ideally as you eat each meal or snack. Trying to remember what you ate the day before is notoriously inaccurate, and even remembering everything you have consumed throughout the day can be difficult. Online calorie trackers can be many calories adrift from actual intake, and this is due to a number of things:

- Inaccuracy in remembering or inputting food intake

- Inaccurate portion sizes input

- Wrong foods chosen from the database

- Inaccurate information in the database.

Researchers at Stanford University tested wearable fitness devices including the Apple Watch, Fitbit Surge, Basis Peak, Samsung Gear S2, Microsoft Band, Mio Alpha 2 and PulseOn. The research on 60 people showed that heart rate information was generally accurate, but the most accurate calorie expenditure was still 27% off the actual expenditure, and the least accurate was 93% off! Calorie content of foods is also inaccurate on many trackers, with the same food items shown with differing calorie contents and often not matching up with the figures in clinical nutrition tables. However, although some researchers have found that people actually gained weight using calorie and/or fitness trackers, they can be a motivating tool to get you moving more and help you to keep track of what you eat.

'Some experts say that the typical 'fad' diet lasts between 3 days and 3 weeks – the same length of time as our differing will power!'

Now it's time to figure out where the hidden calories in your diet are, and choose which foods you want to reduce to give you the weight loss you want.

Finding high calorie foods in your food diary

Once you have a few days' worth of food diary in front of you, look out for the following high calorie foods:

- Full fat dairy products – cheese, butter, cream, milk and yoghurt
- High calorie meals such as take aways, meals eaten out or processed foods
- Sauces and dressings (which are usually based upon oils or fats)
- High fat snacks such as cheese and biscuits, dips or nuts
- Desserts, cakes, biscuits, muffins and other bakery items
- Higher calorie vegetable foods such as olives and avocado
- Alcoholic drinks.

Some foods, such as butter or cream are known to be high in calories, but others may come as a surprise. Check out the chart overleaf to see the approximate calorie count of some foods.

However, not all high calorie foods have to be avoided completely. You need to consider how much of each food you are eating, and how many other high calorie foods you are consuming too. One higher calorie food in a healthy diet is not a problem, as it is the overall calorie intake and calorie expenditure that dictates whether we gain or lose weight. On the other hand, if these foods are your weekly (or even daily) staples, they could be having a significant effect on your waistline. Simply cutting out a couple of glasses of wine in the evening could create enough of a calorie deficit to result in a weight loss of half a pound a week, just from this one change. Foods containing healthy nutrients such as avocado, nuts and olives are good to include in the diet, but you need to make adjustments in your overall diet to be able to include these healthy but high calorie foods. A ketogenic diet (see Chapter 8) is high in fats and yet can provide weight loss, but this only happens when carbohydrate intake is radically low, so it may not necessarily be the high fat foods you choose to reduce, but if you are overweight, something needs to go!

Food	Average calories in a portion
Peanut butter	Spreading peanut butter on a couple of slices of bread or crackers will add an extra 300 calories to a snack attack!
A packet of sandwiches	Many pre-packed sandwiches pack a heavy punch of around 500 calories, providing a substantial amount of the energy most of us need in a day – before you add a packet of crisps and a drink!
Hummus	Dipping your raw vegetables into a dip like hummus can undo your efforts at choosing a lower calorie snack – a large serving can provide well over 300 calories.
Cheese	You may already know that cheese is high in fat and calories, but did you realise that a cubic inch of cheese contains 68 calories, and a cupful of grated cheese over 455 calories?
Potato skins starter with a garlic mayo dip	This tasty starter contains well over 300 calories - before you even tuck into your main meal!
Prawn crackers	Munching away on the free bag of prawn crackers your local takeaway has given you can have you consuming an extra 500 calories on top of your meal!
Double cream	Okay, we all know this is one to avoid on any diet, but it's really worth swapping for Greek yoghurt or fromage frais when you know a helping packs in a whopping 372 calories.
Alcohol	A couple of glasses of wine each evening could be adding 250 calories daily… or 1750 calories over the week…

You may look at your diet and think you can easily reduce your intake by 500 calories a day or you may already be following a reduced-calorie diet or eating healthily, and think there is really no room to reduce your intake any lower. You certainly shouldn't consider reducing your calorie intake below your basal metabolic rate every day (but see information on intermittent fasting in Chapter 8), so if you can't spot ways to easily reduce your calorie intake, and keep it within a healthy range, then you need to look for ways to expend more energy through exercise instead.

However, sometimes we underestimate our calorie intake, or fail to spot habits that are detrimental to successful weight loss. For example, if you add a heaped teaspoon of sugar to tea or coffee, this will add approximately 20 calories to each drink. Five drinks a day is adding 100 calories to your daily intake, and this adds up to 700 calories over a week! Getting used to tea or coffee without added sugar is do-able for most people, and will put a significant dint in your calorie intake. This is also a very good change to make for additional health benefits.

Tips to help you change your diet

- Reducing your daily calorie intake by 250 calories can result in a weight loss of approximately half a pound each week. Do this by…

- Cutting out two large glasses of wine each evening

- Not adding sugar or honey to drinks and cereals

- Cutting out a packet of crisps each day

- Cutting out two biscuits with tea/coffee twice daily

- Reducing cereal portions from 100g to 35g.

Reducing your calorie intake by 500 calories a day can give you a weight loss of 1lb weekly. Do this by…

- Cutting out a bottle of wine each evening

- Cutting out 4 slices of bread or toast with butter or margarine

- Cutting out cracker and dip snacks through the day

- Cutting out the equivalent of 3 – 4 matchbox size chunks of Cheddar or a similar amount of full fat cream cheese

- Eating 150g less starchy carbohydrates such as pasta, rice, potatoes or cereals

- Not having a weekly take away!

The easiest way to adapt your diet without feeling like you are 'on a diet', is to make small changes to lots of aspects of your diet so that you don't miss any one thing too much. By reducing alcohol intake a little, not eating buttered bread with meals, and cutting down on confectionary and take away meals, you can significantly reduce your calorie intake and simultaneously eat a healthier diet. You might note that the changes suggested above mostly involve reducing alcohol or refined carbohydrate foods, which are also known to have a detrimental impact on health too.

Although each dietary change only makes a small difference to your calorie intake, changes like this have 3 benefits:

1 You won't feel like you are on a diet making small changes like this, so you will be able to stick with your new healthy eating regime in the long term

2 In conjunction with other similar dietary adjustments, you will easily and steadily lose weight

3 These changes also promote good health.

Once you have highlighted dietary habits to change on your food diary, there are several ways you can make beneficial changes:

- You could decide to avoid a food/drink altogether

- You might decide to reduce your intake of certain foods/drinks

- You might replace that food/drink item with a lower calorie alternative.

Take a look at the examples highlighted on this food diary and the planned changes below.

'The more changes you make, the bigger the calorie deficit and the greater the weight loss.'

Meal	Monday	Tuesday	Wednesday
Breakfast	Big bowl of granola and semi-skimmed milk. Cup of coffee with semi-skimmed milk and 2 sugars.	Smoothie with 1 banana, 2 handfuls of berries, 300ml almond milk	Pot of yoghurt and fruit. Cup of coffee with semi-skimmed milk and 2 sugars.
Snacks	Biscuits (2) and latte with 2 sugars	Biscuits (2) and latte with 2 sugars.	Biscuits (2) and latte with 2 sugars.
Lunch	Lentil and veggie Soup with bread and butter. Stick of celery and hummus.	Cheese and ham sandwich. Orange juice.	Large jacket potato and tuna with salad.
Dinner	Large portion of lasagna, salad, garlic bread, 2 glasses of Wine, Piece of Chocolate.	Salmon and veg stir fry. Glass of wine.	Steak and and mixed seafood with chips and peas

Food changes to make

Things to avoid altogether

- Stop having bread and butter with meals
- Stop having biscuits mid-morning

Things to reduce

- Reduce cereal portion to 35g
- Have one teaspoon of sugar in coffee instead of two
- Only drink wine two days a week and limit intake to 7 units a week
- Reduce portion size of lasagne and garlic bread but have more salad

Things to replace with a lower calorie alternative

- Change a latte to a normal coffee (mostly water instead of all milk)
- Swap orange juice to water
- Use a handful of spinach instead of half the fruit in the smoothie, and replace almond milk with water

You don't have to change everything in one go – in fact, you're more likely to succeed if you don't make too many changes at once, but allow yourself time to adjust to new eating habits. For example, in the food diary above, the size of the jacket potato hasn't been changed, and chocolate is still on the menu! Make a list of everything you could change, and then decide which things you will change first.

This way of altering your diet will enable you to slowly lose weight. The more changes you make the more weight you are likely to lose, but remember you are in this for the long haul... making smaller changes that you can stick to will enable you to build on your success and stick with it, creating a long term healthy eating plan that suits you.

There are lots of ways to reduce your daily calorie intake. As well as critiquing your usual food intake and making changes there, read on to discover lots of ways that you can adapt your eating behaviour to help reduce energy intake. When each new eating habit becomes a habit that you don't have to think about, choose other changes and add these to your dietary regime.

'Just choose two or three things to adapt and make the changes. Once you are used to these new dietary habits, you are ready to make further changes to your diet.'

Ways to reduce calorie intake

If you have dieted before, you've probably already realised how much psychology is involved in eating behaviour... convincing yourself you've eaten less than you have (or exercised more than you have), persuading yourself that 'The biscuits are low calorie so I can have two', or that an extra bread roll with butter won't matter... your behaviour determines the success or failure of your diet plan. Let's face it – you probably know what you should eat in order to lose weight – it is doing it that is the problem!

Most of us are regularly seduced by the smell, sight and taste of food, causing us to overeat throughout the day. Research shows that we eat more in the following circumstances:

- When we are eating lots of different foods in one meal, especially at buffets or when more than one course is consumed
- When we are doing something else whilst we eat, such as watching television
- If we eat quickly
- If we use larger sized plates that require a greater amount of food to look like a 'plateful' of food.

How many of these circumstances apply to you? Do you eat on the go or whilst watching television? Do you scoff food down quickly and then find yourself looking around for something else to eat? Check out the size of the plates and dishes you use at home – are they larger than other crockery sets you have?

It may be that you don't need to change the types of food you eat at all, but addressing certain lifestyle and eating habits will enable you to lose weight... and making adjustments to both areas of your eating behaviour will pay dividends.

Lifestyle habits that can cause overeating

- Keep tempting foods out of sight! Each time you see the biscuits or chocolate, you will be tempted to eat them. Store foods like this in cupboards that you don't often use. Out of sight, out of mind!
- Avoid having food in easy reach – even nibbling on healthy fruit or nuts is additional calories that you probably don't need.

- Eat light at night! The later you eat in the evening and the bigger the meal, the less likely you are to use up the calories you've eaten. Due to circadian variations in energy expenditure and metabolic pathways, we have reduced thermogenesis and lower metabolic rates, delayed and larger increases in glucose and insulin concentrations in the blood stream after evening meals when compared with meals eaten earlier in the day. Therefore, it is beneficial to try and eat larger meals earlier on in the day, or at least limit calorie and/or carbohydrate intake in the evening meal. Remember, the higher the amount of carbohydrate in a meal, the greater the insulin response, so reducing starchy carbohydrates (pasta, rice, bread or potatoes) in your evening meal is a good idea.

- Get the family involved. If others in the household are eating a healthier diet with you, it becomes easier for you to stick to it.

- Drink plenty of water throughout the day so that you don't mistake thirst for hunger.

- We really don't need to eat three meals a day plus snacks! Don't eat out of habit or just because it's a meal time – you should only eat if you are hungry.

- There is evidence that 'liquid calories' are less satiating than calories from solid foods Limit the amount of high calorie drinks consumed, such as sugary fruit juices, smoothies or lattes.

Eating out

Many people find it relatively easy to eat healthily at home, but encounter calorie control problems when they eat out. Ideally, you should be able to relax and enjoy a meal out, choosing to eat whatever you want to. However, the effects of social eating upon your overall calorie intake will begin to have a detrimental effect upon your energy balance equation if this is a regular event.

Trying to opt for lower calorie options or eat healthily when eating out can be very difficult, as you are basing your decisions upon the menu descriptions, and there are two problems with this:

1 A dish can sound healthy or lower in calories but when it arrives it may be covered in a high fat/high sugar/high calorie sauce or dressing

2 Chefs want their food to taste good, so sugar, salt and fats are used liberally – it is highly likely that most restaurants will use a good deal more sugar, butter, oil, cheese and other fats in their dishes than you would use at home.

Of course, you can always follow well known diet mantras for limiting the calorie damage of eating out...

- Drink still or sparking water instead of juice or alcohol

- Avoid ordering side dishes

- Order salads but hold the dressing or put it on the side

- Avoid snacking on bar and table appetizers such as salted nuts and breadsticks

- Ignore the bread basket!

- Choose soups based upon broths or vegetables rather than cream-based soups

- Choose low calorie vegetable, fish or lean meat options

- Question the waiting staff so that you can make an informed choice of what to eat, and don't be afraid to ask if the chef can modify your meal to suit you by serving sauces and dressings on the side, not adding cheese to a dish, or cream to a dessert.

'Drink less alcohol – it contains almost as many calories as fat!'

Additionally, if you eat out quite regularly, and/or want to be more careful with calorie intake when you eat out, see if any of these tips help:

- Don't feel left out when friends are ordering dessert – order a coffee instead so you have something in front of you to enjoy while they're piling on the calories!

- Share a pudding! Many people feel the need to finish a meal with something sweet – halve the dessert and halve the calories. You'll be doing your pudding partner a favour too!

- Don't starve yourself all day if you're going out for dinner. We are more likely to overeat and choose high fat, high sugar, and higher calorie foods when we're hungry, making it easy to wipe out the 'calorie deficit' you've created during the day.

We really don't need to consume the amount of food that 3 courses provide, and often order a starter, a main meal and a dessert out of habit or for social acceptance (fitting in with what everybody else is doing). Some restaurants offer dishes in starter or main meal size, so you can opt for the starter size, or even order two starters instead of a starter and a main course.

Alcohol

Alcohol can be the ruin of many a good diet! As it comes in liquid form, we often don't consider its calorific value compared to foods, but pure alcohol provides seven calories per gram – just a little less than fats! As a liquid, it's also easy to consume a large volume of it without feeling full, so a couple of glasses of wine in the evenings could be the make or break of your weight loss goals.

But as with any aspect of your diet, you don't need to cut it out completely, unless you want to. Here are some suggestions to help you reduce your alcohol consumption.

- Spritzers last longer than just wine and water down your calorie consumption.

- Alternate alcoholic drinks with mineral water to halve the calories.

- Arrive fashionably late and miss the first round, and if you are drinking at home, start later! If you have made a large dint in a bottle of wine by the time you eat dinner, the wine might not last through the meal, and you'll end up opening a second bottle.

- Don't go out thirsty – the first couple of drinks won't touch the sides! Drink lots of water throughout the day to avoid trying to quench a thirst with the first drinks of the evening.

- Offer to drive.

- Decide to stay within a certain number of alcohol units each week. Work out how many alcohol units you usually drink, and then reduce it. Remember, although it depends upon the alcohol volume of each type of drink, a unit is a generally half a pint of standard strength beer, lager or cider, or a measure of spirits, and a glass of wine is usually two units. It is recommended that we don't exceed 14 units a week for good health, so these are good guidelines to start with if you're currently drinking more than this.

- Have alcohol free days, which is good for the liver too!

Start as you mean to go on

Much of the success of any diet plan comes from being organized and from controlling what is available to eat. Many people comment that they would find it easy to 'diet' if they had a chef producing their food for them – in other words, if you don't have to make the decisions of what food to buy and cook, and didn't have to 'run the gauntlet' of avoiding tasty treats in the kitchen, life would be so much easier! This is why meal replacement diets work for some people – the food choices, decisions and temptations are taken away. But you can gain greater control over what you eat; it just takes a little planning!

Be prepared and take control

- Plan your meals in advance for the week so you know what you will be eating and nothing is left to chance.

- Make a food shopping list and stick to it.

- Don't go shopping if you are hungry. With a low blood sugar level, you will fill your trolley with sugary, refined carbohydrate foods that you wouldn't usually choose, and once you've bought them, you'll eat them!

- Avoid the supermarket aisles that only contain foods you are trying to avoid, so that means ignoring the confectionary and biscuit aisles, with the added bonus that you can reduce the time it takes to do your food shopping.

- Go shopping with a friend or partner who has your best interests at heart – they can step in when your willpower slips.

- If temptation is too much, get someone else to shop for you.

- Shop on-line where you can't see the biscuits, smell the fresh bread or be drawn into buying two for one, when you really only need one....

Summing Up

Okay, so you've bought the food, planned your meals for the week – now you just need to stick to the plan. As long as the meal planning and food shopping have been done with care, you are half way there. Remember...

- Stick to the meals you planned to eat through the week

- Make small changes to your diet that you can stick to

- Employ a mixture of 'cut out', 'reduce' and 'swap to' dietary adjustments

- Think about changes you need to make to how you eat, not just what you eat

- Employ damage limitation when eating out

- Be organised – good organisation with food shopping, meal planning and cooking will pay dividends

- Keep a food diary to keep a check on everything that passes your lips. This is a useful tool to look back over, especially if you fail to achieve the weight loss goals you set for yourself.

5

Calories – Not all calories were created equal!

Most long-term dieters will have counted calories at some point, and a lot of well-known diet plans are based upon calorie content. There's no getting away from the fact that calorie intake balanced against calorie expenditure is a key element of weight control, affecting the amount of adipose tissue (body fat) that you store. However, counting calories can be time-consuming work, and not all calories were created equal! Carbohydrates, protein and fats have different metabolic pathways, and cause the body to require and use differing amounts of energy, which obviously affects the amount of calories you use up and store. This chapter discusses everything you need to know about calories so that you can consider the pros and cons of counting calories in order to lose weight.

What is a Calorie?

A calorie is the amount of energy required to raise the temperature of 1g of water by 1°C. It is the energy currency we use in our bodies – we take food in and break it down, store it, and use it for energy. Caloric energy is trapped in the bonds that hold food molecules together – when we break down (digest) food, we only break it down into smaller units, and much of the energy is still trapped. These smaller units are either:

1 Put to use in the body, retaining the energy

2 Broken down fully to release energy for metabolic activities, general activity or exercise, or

3 Stored, trapping the energy until we need it.

Any carbohydrate not used for energy is stored as glycogen, and any fat not used is stored as adipose tissue. Protein is not stored in the human body. If it is not used for any of its myriad tasks (making enzymes, antibodies, hormones, cell repair etc.), it can be converted into either glucose or ketones and used for energy, or alternatively, excess protein is converted into fat and stored as adipose tissue (body fat). We can store 1600-2000 calories as glycogen energy (stored carbohydrate), giving us enough energy to either get through an entire day relaxing, or providing enough energy for approximately 90 minutes of medium intensity exercise. The amount of glycogen we can store depends upon our body size, which affects the size of our liver and skeletal muscles, and our activity levels, which will affect how much skeletal muscle we have, and how adept at glycogen storage our body is. Most people store hundreds of thousands of calories as adipose tissue.

The word 'Calorie' is actually an interchangeable term used instead of 'kilocalorie' (kcal), which is equal to 1000 calories, but the word 'calorie' is so widely used that we generally only use the term 'kilocalorie' on food labels and nutrition charts, or in nutrition science. The term 'kilojoules' is also seen on food labels; one kilocalorie (Calorie) is equal to approximately 4.2 kilojoules.

Carbohydrate foods such as potatoes, rice, vegetables, fruit, pasta, bread and cereals contain approximately 4 calories per gram.

Protein foods such as meat, fish, eggs, dairy produce or soya contain approximately 4 calories per gram.

Fats such as butter, oils and spreads contain approximately 9 calories per gram.

Alcohol contains approximately 7 calories per gram.

We generalize all the time when talking about foods and calories. For a start, hardly any food is completely carbohydrate, protein or fat, they are usually a combination of these macronutrient food groups. For example, milk may be classed as a protein food but it contains carbohydrate, protein and fat (as well as it's major constituent, which is water); beans are a combination of protein and carbohydrate, and fish is a combination of protein and fat. So when you see a 'calories per 100g or portion' on any food, it is a total of the caloric energy from all the food groups present. Additionally, different types of monosaccharide, amino acid or fatty acid (the individual units that make up the macronutrients carbohydrate, protein and fat) can have slightly different energy yields. For example, 1g of fat from one food may yield 8.6 calories, while 1g of fat from another food may yield 9.35 calories, but we tend to average the energy (calorie) yield from fat molecules as 9 calories per gram. Calorie counts from carbohydrates and proteins are averaged out in the same way.

Most fruit and vegetables have a high water and fibre content, so the caloric energy from the carbohydrates present is usually quite low. 100g of broccoli with a high water and fibre content contain much less energy than 100g of starch-rich potatoes. 100g of avocado, with its high fat content, provides a dense energy source and high calorie content. Foods containing less water or fibre, or with a higher fat content, will tend to be higher calorie foods (as fats provide more than double the amount of energy per gram than carbohydrates and proteins). Fibre is a type of carbohydrate but it is largely indigestible; this means that the energy trapped in the molecular bonds is not released in the human digestive tract, and as a result, much of the fibre proceeds into the stool undigested, having not been broken down to release energy (calories). The bacteria in our gut break down some of the fibre we eat, so it is estimated that fibre provides approximately 2g of calories per gram.

Dietary thermogenesis of each type of macronutrient – the 'net' calorie density!

But even if we know the calorie content of a food, the *net* amount of energy that calories from each type of food provide can differ. This is because each type of food uses up a certain amount of energy during the digestion, absorption and assimilation processes of taking it into the human body. This energy consumption is known as the thermic effect of food, or dietary-induced thermogenesis.

Different types of food use different amounts of energy to be digested and absorbed. Protein takes the most energy – 20-30% of the calories in protein are used up digesting and assimilating it. 5 – 10% of carbohydrate energy is used during the digestive process, and fats use 0-3% of their calories. So if you eat 100 calories from protein, your body uses 20-30 of those calories to digest and absorb the protein, leaving a net calorie gain of 70-80 calories. Carbohydrate would provide a net calorie intake of 90-95 calories, and fat 97-100 calories. This obviously suggests weight loss benefits from eating a higher protein diet. Interestingly, alcohol has a thermogenic effect of 10 – 30%, although alcohol intake tends to be in addition to other nutrients consumed and therefore usually adds to overall calorie intake. The average dietary-induced thermogenesis (energy expenditure) is approximately 10% of the caloric intake of food or drink consumed over 24 hours – this energy is used up in digestion, absorption and immediate storage of nutrients (Westerterp, 2004).

Within the differing thermic effects of foods, storing nutrients as body fat also requires different amounts of energy. The energy cost of storing dietary fats is lower than that of converting protein or carbohydrates into fat. Donato and Hegsted (1985) suggested that dietary fat can be stored as body fat with almost no energy expenditure and, therefore, that dietary fat stored as adipose tissue fat still yields approximately 9 kcal per gram. In contrast, energy is required to store dietary carbohydrates or proteins as body fat – 4 kcal per gram of either of these nutrients yields approximately 3.27 kcal when stored as fat or oxidized for energy.

Researchers have also found that processed foods require less energy to be digested and absorbed than whole foods. In one study (Barr and Wright, 2010) it was found that a processed food meal of the same calorie density as a whole food meal decreased postprandial energy expenditure (the amount of energy used up in digestion/absorption) by nearly 50% compared with the wholefood meal.

Eating processed meals is like eating partially digested foods – they use up to 50% less energy in digestion when compared with whole foods – and that additional energy increases fat storage.

Macronutrient proportions

'Macro challenges' to lose weight or achieve lower body fat levels have become popular amongst some personal trainers and exercisers. Because of the different metabolic roles of proteins, carbohydrates and fats, it is possible that consuming the same amount of calories but with differing macronutrient distribution can affect metabolism, appetite and thermogenesis. Variation in individual responses to different diets suggests that differences may also be associated with specific genotypes.

need2know

Most scientific trials – and possibly anecdotal accounts – illustrate that a higher consumption of protein appears to be beneficial to weight loss and/or reduced weight gain. In an extensive review of the effects of overeating different proportions of carbohydrates, fats and protein, Leaf and Antonio (2017) found that weight gain (fat gain) was less in those over-consuming protein when compared to overconsumption of carbohydrate and fat, between which there was little difference. The main effect of protein upon weight loss is thought to be related to increased satiety – protein takes longer and is more difficult to digest than other types of food, so it keeps us feeling fuller for longer.. High-protein diets seem to be positively associated with weight loss, with favourable body composition and metabolism changes. This is thought to be due to the following:

- Increased satiety, leading to lower calorie consumption

- A higher thermogenic effect, so the *net* amount of energy from each gram of protein is less than other macronutrients

- Improvements in body composition – reducing excess intake of fat and carbohydrate will limit visceral obesity, and in exercising individuals, protein can be used for lean tissue (muscle) development which increases metabolic rate.

Hence the popularity of high protein diets. However, the actual reduction in weight/body fat is due to the reduced calorie intake because of increased satiety, and the increased caloric expenditure through metabolic effects as opposed to energy expenditure through exercise. So it remains feasible that if energy taken in were less than energy expended, the result would still be weight lost, regardless of the proportions of macros consumed. In fact, in their meta-analysis of 32 controlled trials, Hall and Guo (2017) found that both energy expenditure and fat loss were greater with lower fat diets, and studies have also shown weight loss results with ketogenic (high fat, low protein) diets. It may be that the diet that can satiate and control appetite, enabling calorie restriction and energy balance, is the diet that is most successful, and this may be different for each individual.

The Energy Balance Equation

Weight control is based on something called the Energy Balance Equation as shown below.

If energy in = energy out, weight maintenance is achieved.

So, if we take in more calories than we use up, we gain weight, and if our calorie intake is lower than our expenditure, we lose weight. If your weight has been stable for a while, this means you have achieved calorie balance; you are consuming the same number of calories as you are using up. Weight gain indicates that you have been taking in more calories than you need, or are not using up as many calories as you need to. However, your total body weight is affected by water weight, stored glycogen and muscle weight changes which will increase and decrease your body weight more frequently than changes in body fat, so the effect of energy balance is a long term measurement.

It's a balancing act...

You can either reduce your calorie intake or increase your activity levels to lose weight – or, for quicker results, do both. Although calorie counting works for some, not everyone needs to meticulously monitor their energy intake... if you make a few changes in your usual diet to reduce calorie intake and/or do more exercise, you should lose weight, and this can easily be monitored with regular weight loss measurements. It sounds simple doesn't it? It is quite simplistic, but there are many things that affect our food choices and activity levels, and we are also very good at tricking ourselves into thinking we have eaten less, and exercised more than we actually have! Take a look at these common pitfalls that are detrimental to your weight loss efforts...

- Following restrictive diet plans that cannot be maintained for more than a few days – this leads to gorging on foods that you are craving

- Following diets that are too low in calories, leading to low blood sugar levels and higher intakes of food at the next meal

- Not keeping a food diary and forgetting snacks and drinks that have been consumed... a glass of wine, a few chips off someone else's plate, or a handful of crisps...

- Convincing yourself that you have been more active than you really have been, or that you'll go to the gym tomorrow instead – which never happens!

So although the energy balance equation is simple and effective, actually creating a calorie deficit without measuring it can be a little tricky. In order to create a calorie deficit it helps to have a bit more information, such as knowing:

- Approximately how many calories we need each day

- Which foods or drinks are high in calories

- Which foods will satiate us and help to manage food intake

- How to use the thermic effect of macronutrients to our advantage

- How the activity we do each day affects our calorie balance.

Basal Metabolic Rate

Your Basal Metabolic Rate is the number of calories you need each day at rest. If you are quite active you will require more calories; you can take this into account after you have worked out the basic number of daily calories you need. Although it is too time consuming for most of us to weigh the food that we eat and count calories at every meal, it's worth knowing how many calories your body needs each day, as it's a common error to reduce calorie intake too much. Online tools such as MyFitnessPal can be used to log foods eaten, and your intake is shown against your goal, which will be set based on information that you input. If you input that you wish to lose weight, and how much, the calorie intake that is likely to provide this weight loss for you is then shown as your daily calorie goal. Remember though, this is just a guideline, as the number of calories you need is also affected by your height, the amount of lean tissue (muscle) you have, your personal metabolic rate and your activity levels.

Calculating your Basal Metabolic Rate

1 First of all, find your age range in the tables (male or female) below

2 Now multiply your weight in kg by the figure shown for your age

3 Finally, add on the number at the end

To convert your weight in stones and pounds to kilograms follow the guidelines in Chapter Two.

Females

Age	Basal Metabolic Rate
10 – 17	Weight in kg multiplied by 13.4 + 692
18 – 29	Weight in kg multiplied by 14.8 + 487
30 – 59	Weight in kg multiplied by 8.3 + 846
60 – 74	Weight in kg multiplied by 9.2 + 687
75 +	Weight in kg multiplied by 9.8 + 624

Modified Schofield equations. Source: DH 1991)

© Crown copyright. Source: Department of Health.

So, if you were female aged 40 and your weight was 67kg, you would use the shaded boxes and do the following calculation.

67 x 8.3 = 556.1 and then add 846 to give a total of 1402.1 calories.

Males

Age	Basal Metabolic Rate
10 – 17	Weight in kg multiplied by 17.7 + 657
18 – 29	Weight in kg multiplied by 15.1 + 692
30 – 59	Weight in kg multiplied by 11.5 + 873
60 – 74	Weight in kg multiplied by 11.9 + 700
75 +	Weight in kg multiplied by 8.4 + 821

Modified Schofield equations. Source: DH 1991)

© Crown copyright. Source: Department of Health.

'Remember that your BMR is the number of calories you need at your current weight for weight maintenance. If you want to lose weight, you will need to consume fewer calories than this.'

Extra calories for activity and exercise

You can multiply your daily calorie requirement (BMR) by 1.2 to 1.4 to take account of activity during the day. Most of us would not need to adjust our calorie requirement by any more than this, although those doing regular high intensity exercise such as running four or five times weekly might multiply their BMR figure by 1.6 or even 1.8. However, these calculations are based upon active exercisers working at a medium-high intensity level, and it's also worth mentioning here that most of us over-estimate the amount and intensity level of activity we do, so it's unlikely that you will need to adjust your BMR at all if you need to lose weight. Using the earlier example, we would multiply 1402 calories by 1.4 = 1963 calories needed daily. Now you have an idea of how many calories you need each day. The amount of calories that an online or smart device such as a FitBit will show as your daily requirement will be based upon similar equations, depending upon the original BMR calculation that has been programmed in to the device.

The number of calories required is influenced by age, gender, body weight, pregnancy and hormones, such as thyroxin, insulin or adrenaline. Our energy requirement tends to reduce at approximately 2% per decade during adulthood, causing what is often referred to as 'middle-aged spread'. However, this gain in weight is only because of a general decline in lean body mass (muscle). Muscle is denser than fat and is more metabolically active, using up approximately 10 – 15 calories per kg bodyweight/day, in comparison to a kilogram of body fat, which uses up approximately 2 calories/kg/day. Hence, it is favourable to maintain a high muscle mass to maximise caloric expenditure over 24 hours a day, which contributes towards weight control. As weight is one of the variables that affects basal metabolic rate (BMR), the heavier you are, the higher the BMR. As you lose weight, your BMR and therefore your calorie requirements drop.

Don't over do it!

It is a common error to reduce calorie intake too low. This is sometimes done in order to lose weight more quickly and also done when weight loss has stalled, but if you reduce your calorie intake to less than the amount of energy your body needs to function at rest (your BMR) for too long, you are likely to store more fat and muscle is broken down and used for energy. This decreases metabolic rate, and then the number of calories used over a 24 hour period is reduced – this is bad news if you want to lose weight, as you want your metabolic rate to be higher, not lower.

However, it's worth remembering that your calorie requirements are based upon your current body weight: as you lose weight, you require fewer calories as it is easier to move a lighter body around. This is one of the key reasons for the well-known weight loss plateau – we fail to continually adjust our calorie intake as we lose weight. Of course, you can't keep on reducing your calorie intake as the body needs a certain amount of energy and nutrients to function (the BMR you worked out earlier), but this is where regular exercise comes in.

'Watch out for high levels of sugar, salt and additives in reduced fat and reduced calorie foods.'

The pros and cons of calorie counting

The benefit of calorie counting is that if you get it right, you really should be able to control your weight. However, accurate calorie counting requires:

- That you know how many calories you need to consume daily for health, based upon your height, age, gender and current weight

- Accurate portion sizes and weights of food

- The correct brand of food must be input if using websites to calculate your calorie intake

- All food and drinks consumed to be included in your calorie counting (in other words, you have to be honest).

Over time many people get to know which foods are low and high in calories, and can make educated choices about which foods to eat based upon this knowledge. However, calorie counting can be very time consuming, especially if you are being accurate.

Watching out for calories on food labels

But it's not only your nutrient intake you need to worry about... food marketing can be very deceptive, and some so-called 'low calorie' or 'low fat' foods might not be all they seem. If you are relying on food labeling to provide you with accurate information, you have to learn to read between the lines! If fat content is reduced, taste is often affected, so many food manufacturers will add in sugar, salt, sweeteners or flavorings to provide additional flavour. This means that to choose a low fat or low calorie food, you need to check the ingredients list and sugar and salt content as well as fat grams and calories.

Lite or light

'Not all low calorie foods are good for you, and not all high calorie foods are bad for you.'

To use the term 'reduced calorie' on a food, it should contain 30% fewer calories than the standard version. The word 'light' (sometimes spelt as 'lite' on food products) suggests that a food may be lower in calories or fat. To use this term, the food product must be at least 30% lower than other standard products in at least one nutrient or value listed on the nutrition label, for example, lower in fats, sugar or calories, and should state which nutrient it is lower in.

In order to check this out, get used to looking at the 100g list on nutrition labels – this lists how many grams per 100g a product contains, and as most food products show this information, you can easily compare one product with another. To see if a product really is lower in fat or calories, compare it with a standard product – you may be shocked to find the following on 'light' or 'reduced calorie' foods:

- They may be barely lower in fat and/or calories than other products

- They may be lower in fat, but the added sugar for taste has increased the calorie count so that it is no longer a low calorie option

- They may be lower in calories or fat than the same brand's standard version of the same food, but if the standard version is high in calories or fat, the 'light' version may not be low in calories or fat when compared with another brand, or considered to be a low fat or low calorie food.

What is a serving size?

It's also worth checking out the 'calories per serving' information that is shown on some low calorie products. The question is, 'How big is a serving?' If nutritional information per serving size is shown on a food product, the manufacturer must state what a serving size is, and on some products, you may find that the serving size is extremely small. So unless you consume only the amount given as a serving size, you won't benefit from the low calorie intake. For example, a 30g serving of cereal may contain approximately 100 calories, but if you are serving yourself 100g, you are eating over three times the number of calories you may think you are eating.

Low fat products

Many diet products will state that they are low in fat; as fats contain approximately nine calories per gram, the amount of fat in a product is often reduced to lower calorie value. A high fat product contains more than 17.5g of fat per 100g; a low fat product contains 3g or less fat per 100g. It can be misleading when products such as mayonnaise, which are naturally high in fat, are labeled as 'reduced fat' or 'reduced calorie'. Although the fat content may be reduced, the product itself is still classed as a high fat food. Take a look at this example of mayonnaise – the overall fat content is greatly reduced, but the actual fat content of 28.1g/100g means this is still a high fat product.

'Take care when using 'reduced fat' products – they may have a reduced fat content, but could still be high in fat and calories.'

Nutrient content	Calories per 100g	Fat content (g/100g)	Sugar content (g/100g)	Sodium (g/100g)
Normal mayonnaise	724	79.3	0.1	0.24
Low fat mayonnaise	288	28.1	4.6	0.94

Some products based upon fats, such as margarines, may market information such as 'low in saturated fats'. This is likely to be the case, as margarine is not made from saturated dairy fats such as butter, but from polyunsaturated vegetable oils or monounsaturated oils such as olive oil, but all fats, regardless of whether they are saturated, polyunsaturated or mono-unsaturated, contain roughly the same amount of calories per gram, so swapping one type of fat for another will not reduce overall calorie intake, although there is a slightly lower energy content in medium chain fatty acids or medium chain triglycerides, as the slightly shorter fatty acid chains have less energy trapped in the reduced number of bonds.

The downside of low calorie processed foods

When we eat reduced calorie foods, we often give ourselves license to eat more of it because it is lower in calories, often eating so much more that we end up consuming the same number of calories we would have eaten had we consumed the 'full fat' or normal option! One problem with many low calorie foods is that they aren't very filling, and we are likely to eat more of them in order to feel full. Because we are used to a certain satiety level, we continue to eat until we experience a feeling of fullness, which often leads us to consume the same number of calories as usual, even when consuming low calorie foods. Fruits and vegetables don't create this problem because of their natural high fibre content. Fibre makes us feel full, providing the satiety that isn't found with reduced calorie products, although some 'diet foods' now have added fibre to help overcome this and help to fill you up.

Calorie counting versus eating a healthy diet

'Following a healthy diet should involve widening the range of foods that you eat, not reducing it.'

Another problem with very low calorie diets is that the fewer calories you consume, the more difficult it becomes to take in enough of the essential nutrients required for good health – vitamin and minerals, for example. So, ensuring that your diet consists of nutrient-dense foods if you are reducing your overall calorie intake is important. If calorie counting is the only factor that you consider when making food choices, this can sometimes lead to a less than healthy diet, particularly if you have a penchant for biscuits and cakes! There is a wide range of low calorie foods to choose from, but unfortunately, rather than change our diet to one packed with naturally low calorie fruit and vegetables, it can be too tempting to rely upon processed foods labeled as low calorie to reduce energy intake. These foods are often highly processed and contain very little nutritional value. They are also unlikely to satiate you (so you eat more of them), and as mentioned earlier, processed foods can use up only half the usual amount of calories during digestion, which means more calories are available for storage.

So although there are some benefits to counting calories, there are also several considerations, particularly when designing a long term healthy eating plan. It's a good idea to judge a food on its overall merits, considering whether it is healthy and nutritious, rather than just judging how many calories it contains.

Summing Up

Counting calories is just one way to lose weight and maintain a healthy body weight. However, for a healthy long term eating regime, use the information from this chapter to fine tune your energy balance:

- Always consider the Energy Balance Equation

- Calculate your basal metabolic rate to see how many calories you need

- Don't reduce calorie intake below your basal metabolic rate

- 1kg of muscle uses up approximately 10-15 calories per kg bodyweight/day, whereas 1kg of body fat only uses up approximately 2 calories/kg/day

- Read between the lines on food labels

- Make sure low calorie or low fat foods are still healthy options

- Consider the satiety of foods – remember foods with a high protein or fibre content will fill you up and help to prevent overeating and snacking, whereas many reduced calorie and processed foods will make you want to eat more

- Dietary fat can be stored as body fat with almost no energy expenditure whereas energy is required to store dietary carbohydrates or proteins as body fat

- Processed foods require less energy to be digested and absorbed than whole foods, so cut out processed foods for healthy long term weight loss

- 20-30% of the calories in protein are used up during digestion, compared to 5-10% of carbohydrate energy used, and 0-3% of the energy in fats

- Note that the increased satiety, higher thermogenesis and contribution to more lean tissue (muscle) of protein foods will contribute to a better energy balance, tipping the scales in your favour!

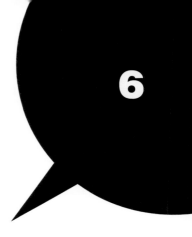

6

Portion size – Just as much to blame!

One thing that many of us need to pay more attention to is the amount of food that we eat, rather than the type of food, where most dietary attention is focused. You can gain weight due to an excess calorie intake from any type of food, not just high calorie or fatty foods, so if you think your diet is healthy, but you struggle to lose or maintain a healthy weight, portion size may be to blame.

Surrounded by temptation

We are constantly bombarded by larger portions of food than we actually need:

- 'Two for one' offers in the supermarket
- 'All you can eat' buffets at restaurants

- Large portion sizes when you eat out
- Large portion sizes at home.

These larger food portions are seen as a bargain, a bonus, good value, or generosity. We don't stop to consider the fact that we don't need, or even really want, the additional food, and once it is bought into the home, or placed upon a plate in front of us, we are likely to consume it.

A study on portion size and calorie intake carried out by Kral et al. (2004) showed that we will automatically eat more food if it is given to us, but still feel satisfied with smaller portions when this is all that is provided. This indicates that we are eating past satiety (fullness) when a greater amount of food or food of higher calorie density is provided.

What happens to the extra food?

Our body can only metabolize and use so much carbohydrate (rice, pasta, vegetables), or protein (meat, fish, eggs) in one go. Excess fats (cream, butter, oils) will simply be stored as adipose fat. Carbohydrates and proteins have many useful roles in the body, but excess that cannot be used (or stored, in the case of carbohydrates) may be converted into fat and stored as adipose tissue (body fat). So you could be eating a fat-free diet (which is not healthy anyway), and still lay down excess body fat if you ate too much carbohydrate or protein. Alcohol follows the same fate: once metabolized in the liver, if it isn't used up for energy, it is stored as adipose tissue. Some fats have important roles in the body, but any excess will be stored as body fat, and much of the saturated fat we eat, which has fewer useful roles in the body, will be stored.

How much is too much?

Protein foods are filling, so we are less likely to over eat these foods. However, carbohydrates, which are digested more quickly, are a different matter. Large servings of cereals, potatoes, pasta and rice are common, and consuming too much in one meal increases the likelihood of the excess carbohydrate being converted into fat and stored. For example, a large 100g portion of cereal may provide approximately 290 calories (without any milk, sugar, yoghurt or fruit added). A 50g portion, which is still quite a large portion, provides 145 calories. Making this change would result in you consuming over 1000 fewer calories weekly – a substantial cut in your energy intake. In addition to this, the smaller cereal portion would require less milk, fruit or whatever is usually added to the breakfast, reducing overall calorie intake even further.

'Study participants consumed 221 fewer calories when offered a smaller meal of lower calorie density, and felt just as full and satisfied as when they had consumed a larger meal of higher calorie density.'

Kral et al, 2004.

However, breakfast should be sustaining enough to provide energy through to lunchtime to prevent snacking, so reduce your portion sizes slowly, and snack on fruit, raw vegetables or nuts mid-morning if you get hungry. It's worth checking out portion sizes of other commonly eaten carbohydrates too, as these are often the foods that we overeat.

- A large (350g, cooked) serving of pasta could weigh in at 467 calories (without the sauce), but a 150g serving provides 200 calories, and a saving of 267 extra calories every time you eat pasta.

- A large (300g, cooked) serving of rice could weigh in at 195 calories (without any sauce), but a 100g serving provides 65 calories, and a saving of 130 extra calories every time you eat rice.

So it's easy to see where those extra calories may be coming from if your portion sizes are a little too large, a little too often! Making changes like this could have a significant effect on your overall calorie intake and also your blood glucose metabolism. Impaired glucose control and insulin resistance – forerunners for Type 2 diabetes – are caused by the intake of excess carbohydrates. Excess carbohydrate intake is also linked to elevated cholesterol and cardiovascular disease, as well as obesity.

Breaking a bad habit

'Eat until you are 80% full.'

Pouring a certain amount of cereal into a bowl every morning, or preparing a certain amount of vegetables for an evening meal is a habit that means you could be consistently preparing more food than you need. Once food is prepared or cooked, it is highly likely that you will consume it all. If your food tastes nice you will want to finish your meal, regardless of whether you feel full or not, and there is also pressure not to waste food and throw it away. Can you see how one action (preparing too much food) is causing another action (eating the food)? The same happens when we go food shopping – if you buy more food than you need, you are much more likely to eat it once it is in the house.

The good news is that simply pouring out less cereal, or peeling fewer vegetables, is somewhat 'removed' from the actual eating process, and is easier to change than trying to exert the will power to stop yourself eating something. If you simply weigh out or prepare less food, you will eat less food. However, you may still need a few additional tips to help, as there is going to be less food – or certainly fewer calories – on your plate.

How to eat less food

The feeling of satiety occurs due to a combination of signals during digestion. These satiety signals are sent to the brain, and are generated in response to:

- The appearance, smell, taste and texture of food
- Expectations about how filling the food or drink is going to be
- Stretching of the stomach
- Hormones released during digestion and absorption of the food or drink.

Hormones tell our brain how much fat is stored in the body, and this affects the feeling of satiety. These signals come together in areas of the brain that control energy intake, and it can take some time after food is first eaten for the full range of satiety signals to reach the brain. We should stop eating once satiety is felt, but there are many things that affect whether we respond to this message from the central nervous system. We are more likely to overeat if food or drink is giving us pleasure (tasting really good), and/or if there is a larger variety of different foods to eat, as in a buffet. Our emotional state and social situation (including who we are eating with and our surroundings, including music, TV, advertising), portion size and food availability all affect how much we eat.

Simple habit can cause us to continue eating past satiety if there is still food on our plate and we are enjoying the food we are eating. The amount of food we eat, and the level of satiety we are used to, are largely habitual, so in order to get past this monumental barrier to weight loss, you will need to know...

1 How to cope with eating less food than you are used to, and

2 How to respond to the satiety message your body is giving you.

Let's take these one at a time.

'Weigh out a 30g serving of cereal and compare it to the amount you normally eat!'

How to reduce your portion sizes and feel fuller

One thing that contributes to our feeling of satiety is the amount of food on our plate. A plate that looks full is less likely to leave us feeling hungry, even if the calorie density is not as high as in a smaller meal. In order to avoid feeling 'short changed', you need to make smaller food portions look like a 'normal' plate full. Here are some tips to help.

- Eat off of smaller plates and dishes so that you don't feel 'cheated' from the outset – making your meal look like a plateful will help to make you feel satiated.

need2know

- Complement your dish with high fibre, lower calorie, less starchy fruit or vegetables. You can gradually reduce the amount of energy-dense pasta, potato, rice or cereal portion of your meal, but fill it out a little with these non-starch polysaccharides, which are higher in fibre and water, and lower in calories. This will help to fill up your plate or dish and increase the size of your meal whilst also reducing calories. Adding a handful of green leaves to meals is a great way to help reduce calorie density of a meal, whilst enhancing the volume of the meal.

- Slow down your eating pace – the faster you eat, the more likely you are to finish your meal before your brain has received any satiety messages. Chewing food for longer will also enhance digestion.

- Sipping water between mouthfuls can help to slow down the pace of your eating. Don't worry, this is unlikely to affect the pH required for digestion of proteins in the stomach.

- Try to include some protein at each meal as proteins make us feel more satiated than carbohydrates or fats.

- Doing something else whilst we eat, like watching TV, takes attention away from our meal, making us more likely to eat quickly, and not notice how much we have consumed. Sit down at the table and be mindful of the food you are eating – enjoy and savor it!

How to respond to the satiety message our body is giving us

- Listen to your body! When you begin to feel full, stop eating!

- Get used to leaving the last couple of mouthfuls on your plate.

- Throw leftovers away immediately so that you don't start eating them later, but note how much food was left, as this is the additional amount of food you have prepared in error. Next time you have this meal, reduce your portion size by this amount to avoid wasted food and temptation to finish the plate.

- Instead of having another serving, refrigerate or freeze left over food for another meal.

'Missing meals or cutting calorie intake too low is a false economy if you overeat at the next meal and over-compensate for the calorie deficit you created earlier.'

Reducing the calorie content of your meal without reducing meal size

Having a full plate or dish of food in front of you will help you psychologically, so that you don't feel like you are 'on a diet', but there are additional benefits to making these dietary changes. As well as being lower in calories, fruits and vegetables tend to contain a very wide range of nutrients such as vitamins, minerals and phytonutrients – plant nutrients that are known to enhance good health. What tends to happen when we are dieting is that as we reduce the amount and range of food we eat, our intake of essential nutrients also reduces, so finding ways to add back in nutrient-dense foods such as these is a bonus. Fruits and vegetables also contain high levels of fibre and water, both essential nutrients that help to reduce calorie intake whilst simultaneously enhancing health. It is the high fibre and water content of these foods that give them a low calorie density, as there are no calories in water and very few that are available to us from fibre, but these nutrients increase the volume of food, helping us to feel full.

What to reduce	What to add in
Reduce your portion size of cereal	Add a handful (portion) of berries, citrus fruits, apple, pear, melon, apricot, kiwi or mango
Reduce your portion of rice	You can add vegetables to the rice whilst it cooks, risotto-style. Pack it out with onions, garlic, frozen peas, peppers and sweet corn. Alternatively, cook the rice separately but add extra vegetables to the other part of your meal, packing out chili, curry or stroganoff with nutrient-dense, low calorie vegetables.
Reduce your portion of pasta	Replace starchy pasta with water-rich aubergines, courgettes, red onions and tomatoes for a lower calorie and tastier Mediterranean style meal with added health benefits! You can even replace all of the pasta with a spiralized 'courgetti', or use carrot, sweet potato or pumpkin instead.
Have fewer potatoes!	Swap potatoes for other vegetables. The bright colours of vegetables such as pumpkin, carrot, beetroot or broccoli denotes the high levels of phytonutrients in these foods, which all contain less starch and fewer calories than potatoes.
Pack out omelettes with vegetables	Add in tomatoes, peppers and onion to fill out an omelette rather than adding other protein foods such as meat or too much cheese.

You could reduce the amount of fish or meat you have on your plate in favour of lower calorie vegetables, however, protein-rich foods like these have a satiating effect upon us, making us feel full for longer, so the reduced calorie intake could be short lived if you begin to feel hungry again soon after your meal. However, your protein portion should be the size of the palm of your hand – even though protein has weight reducing benefits, you can still eat too much of it.

Important note for foodies!

Remember, you are replacing one type of food for another – not simply adding fruit and vegetables to your meals! The plan is to reduce your overall calorie intake, not increase it. If you serve your usual portion of porridge and add fruit to it, this will increase your nutrient intake but also add to your calorie intake. You have to reduce your portion size of starchy carbohydrates, and add some non-starch polysaccharides (fruits or vegetables) to the meal to replace the starchy carbohydrates removed. Adding five tablespoons of different berries to your cereal, or six different vegetables to your pasta (unless in very small amounts!) is also unhelpful – although variety provides a good diversity of nutrients in our diet, having more choice in a meal leads to overeating, so keep it simple. If you increase the proportion or amount of one food on your plate, you have to reduce the amount of another food group. For example, if you added an extra portion of green vegetables to dinner, you should lower the amount of starchy carbohydrate (potatoes, rice or pasta), or sometimes leave out this portion altogether.

Everything in moderation

Although eating a wider range of foods is better for us, it is a common error when preparing food, to cook or prepare a serving size of each food to be eaten, regardless of how many foods are in the meal. A meal of meat, potatoes and peas has three components; a meal of meat, potatoes, peas, carrots and broccoli has five components, so the portions of each, or at least some, of the components, should be lower. However, when preparing food we tend to visualize a 'serving size' of each component on the plate, regardless of how many components are in the meal. If you are preparing a meal with more components to it, you should reduce the amounts of each food in order to limit the overall calorie content.

What is a portion size?

A portion size is approximately the size of the palm of your hand, but how many 'portions' should you have in a meal? A healthy, balanced meal would include the following:

- One portion of protein food (such as fish, eggs, meat or beans)
- Two to three portions of non-starch polysaccharide (fruits or vegetables).
- One to two meals daily *may* contain one small portion of starchy carbohydrates (such as rice, pasta, potato or beans) – this would depend on whether you are following a low carbohydrate diet.

Don't forget that a portion of animal protein (meat, fish, eggs) also contains quite a high amount of fat. Depending on your chosen dietary regime and 'macro-proportions', you may decide to add healthy fats such as olives, nuts, seeds, avocado or vegetable oils to your meal, but if you do, you should be aware of overall calorie content and consider reducing other food groups accordingly.

Current NHS recommendations

The Eatwell Guide illustrates the Department of Health and NHS current recommendations for a healthy balance of foods in the diet. However, recent research has suggested that too many carbohydrate foods may be linked with elevated cholesterol, cardiovascular disease, obesity, insulin resistance and even earlier mortality rates, so many experts recommend consuming a lower amount of starchy carbohydrates than suggested in the Eatwell Guide.

The proportion of macronutrients we should base a healthy diet upon is controversial. A recent large, epidemiological study comparing the dietary intake of individuals in 18 countries with cardiovascular events and mortality showed that higher carbohydrate intake was associated with an increased risk of death (though not with increased risk of cardiovascular disease), and that intake of total fat and each type of fat (including saturated fat) was associated with lower risk of death (Dehghan et al, 2017). This contradicts earlier research that current UK dietary guidelines have been based upon, which is to limit overall fat intake, and saturated fats in particular.

A diverse diet – the pros and cons

Variety and diversity in your diet may be the key to continued good health, but you will have to run the gauntlet of calorie control at every meal. When we are presented with a wider variety of foods, although the range of nutrients is enhanced, the likelihood that we will overeat is higher. This is because a range of different food flavours and textures encourages us to eat more; we are less likely to become bored with one flavour, and the feeling of satiety (fullness) is often interpreted as being related to one food – in other words, we decide we have had enough of one type of food, but will continue to consume other foods. This is experienced when eating out – we may feel 'full' and would not choose to order another plate of lasagna, for example, but will gladly eat dessert.

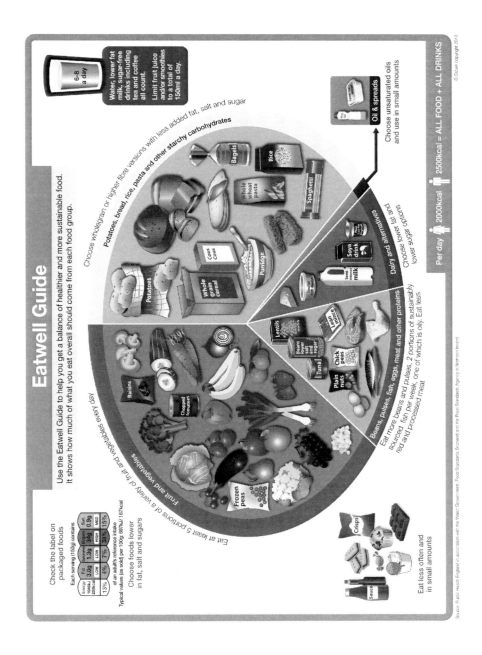

Therefore, when replacing some of your calorie-rich foods with other foods, don't add too many different foods to a meal – if you are replacing some of your rice/pasta/cereal/potato with fruit or vegetables, just add a small amount of each fruit or vegetable; if you are omitting your starchy carbohydrate from a meal, replace it with two portions of non-starch polysaccharides.

Rice should be weighed before cooking as it absorbs so much water during the cooking process and vastly increases its weight, so dry weight of rice will always look like a much smaller portion than it will be on the plate. You will find that raw fruit and vegetables weigh quite heavy due to their natural water content, so replacing 50g of rice with, for instance, carrot, would mean adding only a quarter of a large carrot. However, 89% of carrots are water weight and carry no calories, whereas only 11.4% of white rice is water weight and the rest of the weight is calorie dense nutrients, so you can add a greater weight or volume of the non-starch polysaccharide foods and still create a calorie deficit.

This table shows the relative water, fibre, nutrient and calorie content of various foods. There are no calories in water, so the greater the amount of water in 100g of a food, the lower the overall calorie content is. All foods are uncooked to compare the actual calorie content of 100g of rice compared with carrots, oats compared with blackberries, and potatoes compared with broccoli. You can see that because fruits and vegetables contain so much water and fibre weight, you could double the weight of these foods to the amount of starchy carbohydrate you have removed, and still have a lower calorie intake.

	Water weight	Protein (4 calories per gram)	Fat (9 calories per gram)	Carbohydrates (4 calories per gram)	Fibre	Overall calories per 100g
White rice	11.4	7.3	3.6	85.8	0.4	383
Carrots	89.8	0.6	0.3	7.9	2.4	35
Ready Brek	8.3	11.6	8.3	65.4	8.0	366
Blackberries	85	0.9	0.2	5.1	3.1	25
Potatoes	79	2.1	0.2	17.2	1.3	75
Broccoli	88.2	4.4	0.9	1.8	2.6	33

Source of information: McCance and Widdowson's 'The Composition of Foods Integrated Dataset', 2015.

Why starchy carbohydrates are the foods to limit

Protein foods provide satiety and a metabolic advantage when considering net calorie contribution to energy balance (i.e. more of their energy is used up during digestion and absorption than other nutrients), although the portion size of a protein food should still be limited to approximately the palm of your hand. You will notice that most suggestions to reduce portion size are based upon reducing starchy carbohydrates. If the protein portion of the meal is measured, then the fat content will also usually be limited, as this is where most fats occur, within the meat, fish, eggs or dairy part of our meals. Of course, added fats such as avocado, oils, butter or nuts add calories to a meal and the amount eaten should be considered carefully. Swapping starchy carbohydrates for non-starch polysaccharides is a perfect swap as the vegetables or fruits provide the fibre and nutrients lost in the starchy carbs, whilst simultaneously reducing calorie intake and also having a beneficial impact on blood glucose and insulin levels. Limiting starchy, sugary and refined carbohydrates will have the most profound effect upon insulin metabolism, and as it is becoming increasingly clear that hyperinsulinaemia and insulin resistance play a major role in the development of obesity, diabetes and cardiovascular disease, this is the food of choice to limit.

'For an easy and nutritious swap, replace starchy carbohydrates with a handful of rocket or watercress - this is a great calorie saver.'

Summing Up

Portion size is the root of the problem for many dieters, and although it is always important to consider what you are eating, the amount consumed is of equal value.

For a weight loss plan that works for life, keep an eye on your portion sizes. Remember...

- Prepare less food to begin with – you can always have a snack later if you haven't had enough to eat, but if you prepare too much, it's likely you will eat it whether you need it or not

- Fill up your plate with lower calorie foods such as vegetables – the increased size of the meal will make you feel fuller

- Reducing starchy carbohydrates will help create weight loss, and also offer multiple health benefits.

- Include some protein at each meal

- Eat slowly – and stop eating once you feel full

- Remember, satiety is specific – a smorgasbord of food will result in a higher calorie intake.

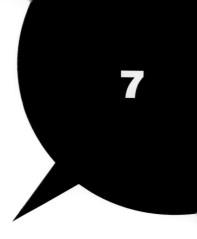

7

Weight Loss through Exercise

Weight loss is most successful when healthy eating is combined with regular exercise. Energy expenditure is one half of the energy balance equation, and, as well as keeping you fit and healthy, the more active you are, the more calories you can consume without gaining weight. However, if the very mention of exercise has you breaking out in a (cold) sweat, the likelihood is that you've just not found an activity that suits you yet. Let's explore how you can lose weight by using up more calories through activity and exercise.

This chapter is for you if…

- You find it difficult to find ways to reduce your current calorie consumption
- You would prefer to keep some 'treats' in your weekly diet and use activity and exercise to create a calorie deficit

- You want to make exercise a regular part of your healthy living regime, or

- You want quicker results by reducing calorie intake and simultaneously increasing calorie expenditure.

There are many ways of using up more calories throughout the week. Regular exercise is the best way to use up large amounts of energy, but increasing your activity throughout the day can also help. Even if you exercised for an hour daily, there are still another 23 hours in each day (15 if you deduct 8 hours for sleeping!) during which you can help yourself to lose weight. Here are some ways in which you could fit extra activity into your daily routine. As with the tips to reduce calories, choose the options that will suit you the most, as you'll be more likely to stick with them.

Fitting more activity into your life

- Use the stairs rather than the lift – especially if you work or live somewhere with stairs and can make this a regular calorie burner.

- Don't send e-mails to office colleagues – bring back the art of conversation and walk to their desk to give them a message.

- Don't drive around car parks until a space right next to the door is free – park further away and walk. Even better, leave the car at home!

- Get off the bus, tube or train a stop early.

- Walk the children to school.

- Walk to the shops instead of sending someone else or using the car.

- Take up an active hobby such as dancing or gardening.

- Take the dog (or other people's dogs) for a walk.

- Don't put the housework off – it may be boring, but vacuuming, dusting and even ironing can all notch up reasonable calorie expenditure.

Exercise

Nothing can beat the benefits of regular exercise for reducing body fat levels and helping you to maintain a healthy body weight. Although many people begin exercising to lose weight, if you choose an exercise that you enjoy, you'll feel healthier and fitter, and also enjoy the social benefits that many types of exercise offer. Weight loss often just becomes an added bonus!

How much exercise do I have to do?

If you plan to lose 1lb a week, you need to create a calorie deficit of approximately 500 calories a day – but how long would you need to exercise to do this? It depends on how much effort you put in, and which type of exercise you choose to do. The higher the intensity, the more calories you use up, so you can exercise for a shorter period of time if you are prepared to work harder. For example, you would need to walk at a fast pace for almost twice the time it takes to expend around 500 calories in a 45 minute run.

Of course, the amount of calories you use up is individual; your weight, body composition and fitness level all affect how much energy you utilise. But as a guideline, here are some examples of workouts that would use up approximately 500 calories…

- 45 minutes on a step machine in the gym
- Just over an hour playing a reasonably hard game of tennis
- Three to four hours of golf (without the buggy!)
- One hour of cycling.

'The most important thing about exercise is to make it a regular occurrence!'

How hard do I need to work?

Most of us exercise well within our comfort zone at a level that feels comfortable, without getting out of breath or sweating too much. However, this fails to give us a 'training effect'. Scales of perceived exertion can be used to determine the intensity level of exercise (how hard someone is working). On a scale of 1 – 10 of perceived exertion, we often remain below 6. To really make a difference, you should exercise at a perceived exertion rate (RPE) of 7 – 8.

The Talk Test is used in the health and fitness industry to help exercisers measure their exercise intensity level. If you can have a full conversation with someone without getting breathless, you're unlikely to be exercising at a high enough intensity to create a training

'The more you weigh, the more calories you use when you exercise, so as you lose weight you will use fewer calories during your exercise session. This is one of the main reasons for weight loss slowing down, and means you have to work harder to use up enough energy to continue to create a calorie deficit.'

effect – you're taking it easy! However, you should be able to speak a sentence or two – if you can't say anything, your intensity level is too high to be maintained for long, certainly not throughout an endurance activity such as swimming or running.

It is essential that you continue to push yourself as you become fitter and lose weight. As your body becomes used to the exercise, the activity becomes easier to do. This adaptation, combined with any weight loss, means that you are using fewer calories during the same workout, and the exercise will begin to contribute less to your weight loss goal. Exercising for longer, changing the exercise session, or increasing the intensity will ensure that the exercise you do remains effective.

How long do I need to exercise for?

The American College of Sports Medicine is an authority on the effects and benefits of exercise. Their recommendation for all healthy adults is as follows:

- Do at least 150 minutes of moderate-intensity exercise per week.

- This can be either as 30-60 minutes of moderate-intensity exercise (five days per week) or 20-60 minutes of vigorous-intensity exercise (three days per week).

- Multiple shorter sessions (of at least 10 minutes) are acceptable to complete the desired amount of daily exercise.

The ACSM also recommend that adults should do some strength, flexibility and functional fitness training each week:

- Adults should train each major muscle group two or three days each week using a variety of exercises and equipment.

- Adults should do flexibility exercises at least two or three days each week to improve range of motion.

- Functional fitness training is recommended for two or three days per week, involving motor skills (balance, agility, coordination and gait).

The longer you exercise for, the more calories you will use up. As we use up our stores of carbohydrate (which generally last for approximately 90 minutes of medium to high intensity exercise), we begin to use more fat, so exercising for longer results in more fat being used up. For exercise sessions longer than 40 minutes duration, work out at a medium intensity to maximize fat-burning potential. If you have less than 40 minutes available for a workout, you will need to exercise at a higher intensity for the same caloric expenditure. Try to exercise at a RPE of 8.

So, the less time you have available to exercise, the harder you'll have to work to burn the same amount of calories.

What type of exercise is best?

Cardiovascular exercise

Cardiovascular exercise is any activity that makes the heart and lungs work harder – the type of activity that involves large body movements and gets you out of breath. Here are some examples of popular cardiovascular (aerobic) exercise:

- Walking and power walking
- Jogging and running
- Swimming
- Cycling
- Swimming
- Fitness classes
- Dance classes
- Rowing
- Step and cross training machines

As cardiovascular exercise uses large muscle groups, this is the type of exercise that uses more calories, so you need to include some types of cardiovascular exercise in a weight loss routine every week.

Weight bearing exercise burns more calories

Although any type of exercise is a good thing, there are some types of exercise that are better then others as far as calorie expenditure is concerned. These tend to be the higher intensity cardiovascular exercises such as running, but exercises where you are supporting your body weight will use up more energy than exercises where your body weight is supported. For example, cycling and rowing are classed as non-weight bearing exercises as your body weight is supported by being seated. Although these types of exercise are still beneficial, you have to work harder at them to use up the same number of calories you would expend in a weight bearing exercise over the same length of time. When you are swimming your body weight is supported by the buoyancy of the water, making this a non-weight bearing exercise. However, you do have to propel yourself forwards through the water, so this helps to increase the intensity of swimming.

Take a look at the chart below that gives approximate calorie expenditure per hour for various activities. The weight bearing activities shown in the shaded boxes use up more calories than the non-weight bearing types of exercise. All figures are approximate as your calorie expenditure depends upon your weight, height, age, gender and body type.

'Weight bearing exercises use more calories than seated exercises, and the weight bearing on the bones helps to improve bone density.'

Activity	Approximate calories/hour
Running (7.5 miles per hour)	697
High impact aerobics	414
Rowing at moderate intensity	365
Cycling (10 miles per hour)	305
Swimming (recreational)	250

Information from www.weightlossresources.co.uk

This doesn't mean that you shouldn't swim, cycle or row, it just means that you have to work harder at these activities, or do them for longer, to make them as effective as weight bearing activities.

High intensity interval training (HIIT) and moderate Intensity continuous training (MICT)

HIIT is just a combination of interval and circuit training, usually using different workout stations to target different muscles and increase exercise variety. It is a popular workout choice as it tends to be fairly short in duration (30 – 45 minutes) and is effective for weight and body fat loss. A review by Wewage et al in 2017 reported no significant difference in body fat reduction between those engaged in HIIT and MICT, although both were effective in reducing body fat, and HIIT required approximately 40% less time. Thivel et al (2018) also found that HIIT improved aerobic fitness, body composition and cardio-metabolic risk factors, but data was insufficient in their meta-analysis to determine whether it is more effective than lower intensity exercise.

Maillard et al (2018) analysed 39 studies involving 617 subjects and found that HIIT significantly reduced total fat, abdominal fat and visceral fat mass, and that running was more effective than cycling in reducing total and visceral fat mass (a finding also reported in other studies). High-intensity (above 90% peak heart rate) training was more successful in reducing whole body adiposity, while lower intensity training had a greater effect on changes in abdominal and visceral fat mass.

Whether HIIT is more effective at reducing body fat levels than other forms of exercise is not important – the key thing is that any type of exercise will be helpful in increasing energy expenditure and reducing body fat.

Weight training

Although you may be seated during many weight training exercises in the gym, it is considered a weight bearing exercise because of the resistance applied against each muscle worked. This, combined with the training effects of weight training, make the gym a good option for weight loss.

It is a common misperception that weight training will increase body weight. However, although weight training may increase the amount of lean tissue (muscle) you have, and may therefore increase your overall body weight by a little, the overall effect will reduce body fat levels, as the more muscle you have, the higher your metabolic rate is. This means that you will use up more calories, whatever you are doing, over a 24 hour period. Gaining lean tissue helps to turn your body into a fat-burning machine!

Unless you follow a body building routine lifting heavy weights you won't build large muscles, and most weight training programmes will tone up the muscle that you have, tightening muscles and shaping your body. This in itself will make you look and feel slimmer, so it's a good idea to include one or two weight training sessions a week in your fat loss exercise programme in conjunction with some calorie-burning cardiovascular exercise.

The best exercise for weight loss

Interval training is very effective for weight loss – this is when you work hard for a set time, then exercise at a lower intensity for a time (altering the timings as you become fitter). Working harder for short spurts enables you to exercise harder than you usually would, as you only stay at this level for a short period of time. During the higher intensity phases you use up more calories than normal, but the lower intensity phases (when you return to your 'normal' exercise intensity level) allow you to recover. Doing an entire workout at the higher intensity level is unrealistic, but adding spurts of higher intensity will burn more calories and increase your fitness levels. You can incorporate interval training into many different types of exercise.

'For every extra pound of muscle you put on, your body uses around 50 extra calories a day. In one study, researchers found that regular weight training boosts basal metabolic rate by about 15%. This is because muscle is 'metabolically active' and burns more calories than other body tissues even when you're not moving.'

Juliette Kellow, Weight Loss Resources.

- Jogging – Jog for a minute then walk for a minute. As you become fitter, increase the time you spend jogging, and decrease the time you spend walking.

- Cycling – Cycle at a faster speed for two minutes, then slow down for a minute. As you become fitter, increase the faster cycling time, or add in some hills, which also heighten intensity.

- Swimming – Swim one length quickly then swim back at your normal pace. Try to gradually increase the ratio in favour of faster lengths, so progress from a ratio of 1 slow: 1 fast to 1 slow: 2 fast, 1 slow: 3 fast and so on. You can also combine higher intensity swimming strokes such as front crawl or butterfly with lower intensity breaststroke.

Activity trackers

Before there were smart watches and wireless activity trackers, pedometers blazed the way, counting the number of steps walked or calories burned. Whatever type of device you use, it can be a good tool to help increase the amount of activity you do just by moving around more, and you can set yourself a daily step or calorie goal. In the run-up to the 1964 Tokyo Olympics, a company came up with a device called a Manpo-Kei, which translates as '10,000', 'steps', and 'meter'. This early pedometer was based on the work of Dr Yoshiro Hatano, who felt that the health of the nation would be improved if everyone increased their daily steps from 4,000 to around 10,000 (an increase of 6000 steps). Fitbit users will know that walking for 6000 steps uses up approximately 500 extra calories... and if you were to create an energy expenditure of an additional 500 calories daily, this represents a fat loss of 1lb a week, as there are 3500 calories in a pound of fat. That, apparently, was how the '10,000 steps a day' regime was born, and is still programmed into many devices as the daily goal.

If this is much more than you currently do in a day, it may be an unrealistic target. Instead, find out how many steps you do in a typical day, and then set a target to increase your steps by (for instance) 10%, or add on an additional 300 steps. Once you are achieving your target steps each day, set a new goal to increase it again.

Getting started and sticking with it

It can be really difficult to begin – and stick with – a regular exercise regime. How many times have you begun to exercise and then stopped – or maybe never got started in the first place?! However, there are a number of psychological tools you can use to create a regular exercise habit and achieve your weight loss goal.

Dissociation

For many people, being out of breathe, feeling hot and sweaty, and exercising at a high intensity is not an enjoyable experience, and the only way to get through it is by doing something that takes your mind off of exercise. This is called exercise dissociation. Take a look at these common ways of 'switching off':

- Listening to music whilst you exercise

- Watching TV or listening to music in a gym

- Chatting with a friend whilst you exercise.

Dissociation takes your mind off of the exercise you are doing and relieves boredom and exercise discomfort.

Exercising with others

One of the most successful ways to stick with regular exercise is to exercise with other people. This is for a number of reasons:

- It can take your mind off the exercise

- It can relieve boredom

- It can make the exercise more enjoyable and sociable

- You are less likely to miss an exercise session if you are letting someone else down

- There may be an element of friendly competition

- A bit of morale support helps!

'Up to 80% of people do not have the 'self management' skills to continue with regular exercise without some sort of support system, explaining why many of us stop and start exercise many times over the years.'

Enjoy exercise!

It is essential that you find something that you enjoy doing – if you don't enjoy it, you won't keep it up. There are many different reasons for exercising, which can be split into extrinsic and intrinsic factors. Tick off any of the examples below to help you decide whether your exercise motivations are, or have been, intrinsic or extrinsic.

Intrinsic (you gain satisfaction from exercising itself)

☐ I enjoy the way regular exercise makes me feel

☐ Regular exercise makes me feel healthier

☐ Exercise energizes me

Extrinsic (you are exercising for a benefit other than the exercise itself, for example, to lose weight)

☐ I need to exercise to lose weight

☐ I have to exercise to look better

☐ I should start running to get in better shape

The difference is that extrinsic factors are less likely to help us stick with exercise in the long run. If you exercise because you feel you have to, ought to or should do, this is shaky ground for a long term exercise habit. If, however, you exercise because you enjoy it, or you like the way regular exercise makes you feel, these intrinsic factors are linked with a healthy, long term exercise habit which will support long term weight loss.

How will I know what type of exercise I enjoy?

In the same way that we choose our hobbies or careers, there is an activity or type of exercise out there for everyone… you just need to figure out what suits you! You may need to think back to the last time you exercised regularly (which might have been at school), and try to remember what activities you enjoyed... was it team sports, competitive sport or more social/fun activities?

Various studies have linked exercise success to different personality traits – if you choose a type of exercise that suits your personality, you're more likely to enjoy it, and if you enjoy it, you'll stick with it. See if you can spot your personality and then try out the suggested activities for your type.

'Some research has shown that 90% of us prefer to exercise with others, and we are up to 22% less likely to stop exercising if we exercise with other people.'

Spot yourself…	Try one of these…
Competitive	Squash Tennis 10 km competition runs Triathlons
Sociable	Fitness classes (anything from yoga to HIIT) Running or walking clubs Get involved in a squash or tennis league Swimming clubs or aqua aerobics
Self motivated	Go to the gym and set weekly goals Running, cycling or walking alone You'll be able to go swimming and just complete lengths of the pool
You have a sense of adventure	Mountain biking Water sports Hill walking Diving – join your local sub aqua club
Do you have an aggressive nature or need to let off steam?	Boxercise classes Kickboxing or other martial arts Crossfit training Running

The most important thing is that you enjoy what you're doing, so try a few different things and see what works for you.

Finding time to exercise

The factor quoted most often as a reason for not exercising is lack of time. Exercise takes a back seat to almost everything else in most people's lives, but we often over-estimate how much time is needed to fit in an exercise regime that will make a difference. Remember, every bit counts – even if you only exercise for 20 minutes it might use up an extra 100 calories, will increase your metabolic rate for a while, and help you to get into the habit of exercising.

Think about when you could exercise...

- An early workout before breakfast
- During the day
- In a lunch break

- After work in the evening

- At the weekend.

Although this may seem fairly obvious, it's worth taking time to plan when you will exercise, and organising your day around it. Write it in your diary or on the calendar and begin to book other things around the exercise, rather than trying to fit exercise in around everything else.

'Having an "all or nothing" attitude to exercise often results in 'nothing' being done. If you haven't got enough time for a one hour workout, just do two shorter workouts!'

Benefits of an early morning workout

- Working out first thing means that regardless of how your day turns out, you have already exercised. This is a good option if you have a busy schedule, or if you are likely to put off exercise.

- Early morning exercise is a great energizer, setting you up in a great frame of mind for the rest of the day, and can help you to stick to your healthy eating plans.

- Early morning exercise can be an effective 'fat burning' workout as you will have less stored carbohydrate available and will use more fat for fuel.

Lunchtime exercise benefits

- Research shows that exercise at lunchtime improves focus, concentration and effectiveness during the afternoon when energy and concentration levels usually drop.

- The sociable aspect of exercising with work colleagues will increase your enjoyment of exercise, and once you're in the habit of going to the gym or going for a walk at lunchtime, you are likely to stick with it.

- Exercising during the day gets the workout done before you relax at home in the evening, when it is notoriously difficult to find motivation to go and exercise.

Exercising in the evening

- Early evening is the time when our circadian cycle is at it highest, making 4pm to 6pm the most effective time for exercise.

- You are less likely to have pressing engagements that limit exercise time, so you can spend longer exercising if you want to.

Weekends and days off are typically a time when, although there is more time for exercise, the time is often spent doing other things. Try to do different types of activity with friends or family, which will help you to use up more energy...

- Go for a walk
- Go swimming
- Go cycling
- Do an activity such as horse riding or ice skating
- Play tennis or badminton with family or friends.

Goal setting

Setting exercise goals can also help you to stick with regular exercise, and can be a better type of goal than a weight loss goal. Weight loss goals are based up body measurements, which can be unpredictable and de-motivating when we don't get the results we want. However, if we measure the exercise we do in order to lose weight we have more control over the outcome and are likely to be more motivated by the results along the way.

For example, you might decide that you will exercise twice weekly, note down your exercise sessions as you do them, and tick off that achievement at the end of the month. An even better goal is to plan a set number of workouts per month so that you can play 'catch up' in case you miss a workout, and the goal is not lost immediately. Planning to complete a set number of exercise minutes is even better, and your goal should be based upon current activity levels and realistic aims, but also pushing yourself a little.

Get a personal trainer

If all else fails and you simply can't motivate yourself to exercise regularly, why not get a personal trainer? It is often less expensive if you buy multiple sessions, and having one session weekly may motivate you to exercise on your own or with a friend between sessions. Plus, you'll have the benefit of having a professional who will note measurements, help you to set goals and monitor your progress in addition to getting the most out of you in each exercise session!

'Measuring weight loss is an outcome goal based upon the results of weeks of dieting and exercise, whereas measuring the amount of exercise done is a process goal. For increased success, measure the journey rather than the outcome.'

Summing Up

So, taking all that into account, a successful exercise plan for weight loss will look like this:

- Choose a type of exercise that you enjoy
- Unless you are self motivated, plan how you can exercise with a friend or group
- Set yourself an exercise goal that you can either measure each week, and/or will measure in 4 to 6 weeks time
- Choose weight bearing and higher intensity activities that will use up more calories
- Using an activity tracker can help motivation and exercise frequency
- Try to add some spurts of higher intensity into your exercise session, and keep your overall rate of perceived exertion (RPE) at around 7 – 8.

If you're really keen to lose weight, reducing your calorie intake and increasing your calorie expenditure will obviously create a bigger calorie deficit, as you take in less and use up more energy. Just make sure you're eating enough to provide energy for your exercise sessions!

8

A review of popular weight loss diets

We have already established that to create weight loss, you have to create a calorie deficit. This can be done in lots of different ways, which explains the myriad of diets available – but which ones are most likely to work long term? Basing your diet on quick fix supplements or restrictive diets is neither healthy nor effective. To understand how you will lose weight and keep it off, you need to know a little about how the human body works, so in addition to reviewing some popular diets this chapter explores the effects on metabolism in the human body.

Fasting

Fasting has become more popular in recent years, for both weight loss and health benefits. In particular, fasting on one or two days a week, or extending the overnight fast by eating the evening meal earlier, not having breakfast (the 'break' of the fast) or breakfasting later in the morning, are popular regimes.

Types of fasting

16:8

This involves daily fasting for 16 hours, or eating all of your meals within an 8 hour window. For example, breakfast is delayed until 11am and dinner finished by 7pm.

20:4

Fasting can be adapted to create an even shorter eating window and a longer fast, for example, missing breakfast and lunching late, only eating a couple of meals between 2pm and 6pm, or one large meal.

5:2 / The Fast Diet (Intermittent fasting)

These diets aren't really fasting, but reducing calorie consumption to 500 calories for women/600 for men on two days a week, eating as you normally would on the remaining 5 days. This reduction in calorie intake from the NHS guidelines of 2000 for women/2500 for men creates a caloric deficit of approximately 1500/2000 on each 'fasting' day, and an overall reduction in calories of 3000 – 4000 each week, which is roughly equivalent to the energy in one pound of stored fat (3500 calories). Hence, this regimen should result in a steady weight loss of approximately 1lb or half a kilogram weekly.

Another benefit of intermittent fasting is that you are only reducing your calorie intake for two days in a week, so you may be able to stick with this eating plan if you have failed with other diets. Researchers found that, contrary to initial presumptions that dieters would overeat after the fasting days, people generally just ate what they would normally have eaten. Obviously, if you gorge on foods in the remaining five days and offset the calorie reduction, you won't lose weight. During short (day long) 'fasts', such as those on the 5:2 diet, unless only very little carbohydrate and sufficient fat is consumed, ketosis will not necessarily become the predominant source of energy as it does on a ketogenic diet.

Although this way of eating isn't necessarily improving the quality of the diet – there are no restrictions or guidelines on which foods provide the reduced or usual calorie intakes – any reduction in body weight does provide health benefits.

Health benefits of fasting

Fasting has been practiced for millennia, but we are only now beginning to understand the adaptive cellular responses that reduce oxidative damage and inflammation, and boost cellular protection – in short, fasting can delay the ageing process. It reduces obesity, hypertension, asthma, and rheumatoid arthritis. Studies of intermittent fasting show reduced blood pressure and cholesterol levels, and improved insulin sensitivity; in some cases it facilitates a reversal of type 2 diabetes. Even in studies where participants have fasted intermittently but controlled calorie intake so that no weight is lost, insulin sensitivity improved.

Harvie and Howell (2016) illustrated that intermittent energy restriction caused greater improvements in insulin sensitivity and comparable reductions in inflammatory markers when compared with continuous energy restriction. A 2014 review found that intermittent fasting regimens demonstrated body weight reductions of 3–8% after 3–24 weeks in comparison to energy restriction diets, which demonstrated 4–14% reductions in weight after 6–24 weeks. Both weight loss strategies yielded comparable reductions in visceral fat, fasting insulin, and insulin resistance.

A 2018 study found no difference in the time it took to achieve a 5% weight loss between participants who were on an intermittent fasting regime, compared with those on continued energy restriction. Both diets reduced insulin levels, but the intermittent fasting diet participants had lower blood lipid levels after eating.

Although there are some health benefits to longer term fasting, if fasting continues past a few days, the metabolic rate can be affected, as energy expenditure adapts to cope with the reduced caloric intake (adaptative thermogenesis). Resting metabolic rate increases with overfeeding, but can decrease by as much as 20% during food restriction. However, this may be predominantly as a result of lean muscle loss, so limiting the loss of lean tissue by consuming ample calories as fat to enter into ketosis, which conserves muscle, or exercising to promote lean tissue maintenance, may offset this reduction in metabolic rate. Whether an ample amount of protein and fat can be consumed will depend on the type of fast, and exercise will be dependant upon energy levels.

Metabolic effects of fasting

If a meal is missed, blood glucose levels drop. The resulting secretion of the hormone glucagon stimulates the breakdown of glycogen (stored carbohydrate), which releases glucose into the bloodstream. This glucose provision will supply the body for between 12-24 hours if glycogen stores were originally sufficient. When a fast is continued and glycogen stores have been largely used up, the human body can manufacture glucose from non-carbohydrate sources such as glucogenic amino acids, lactic acid and glycerol. The enzyme lipase also breaks down stored fats (triglycerides) into glycerol and fatty acids – the glycerol is turned into glucose via gluconeogenesis, and the fatty acids are partially oxidized, forming something called ketones (acetone, acetoacetate, and beta-hydroxybutyrate). We usually form some ketones in the liver, but the levels rise as our carbohydrate or caloric intake reduces.

The formation of ketones provides the fuel that is needed and reduces the break down of protein and/or muscle tissue. So energy during a short fast will be taken mostly from glycogenolysis (breaking down and using glycogen (carbohydrate) stores), gluconeogenesis (making new glucose from proteins, glycerol and lactic acid), and the breakdown of adipose tissue (fat). In prolonged fasting or very low calorie intakes, muscle tissue may be broken down for energy, which is not conducive to good weight loss as this will reduce your overall metabolic rate.

Ketosis

During prolonged fasting or starvation, the hypothalamus secretes a hormone called ghrelin, which increases appetite and also stimulates the pituitary gland to release Growth Hormone. Growth Hormone 'switches off' the body's uptake and use of glucose and switches it to oxidising fats for energy, at which point, ketones, rather than glucose, become the mainstay of energy production. After around three days of starvation, fasting, or very low carbohydrate intake, roughly a third of the brain's energy is supplied by ketones, which also supply the heart. We produce ketones in the liver all the time, but the action of 'going into ketosis' denotes when the body has a very low carbohydrate intake and virtually no stored carbohydrate, and must make more ketones to provide energy.

What about 'grazing' through the day?

Fasting is a contradiction to the well-known recommendation to 'eat regularly to balance blood sugar levels' or 'graze through the day'. It has previously been thought that eating regularly keeps blood glucose levels from dropping too low and prevents overeating from hunger. In good health, the hormone glucagon should stimulate breakdown of stored carbohydrate to release glucose into the blood stream, therefore keeping blood glucose levels fairly stable – and of course we also have many thousands of calories of energy stored as fat to use too! Added to these mechanisms the ability to form glucose from other sources (gluconeogenesis), and you can see that a healthy body has the tools to go without food, or with less food, for a significant period of time. Of course, some people do experience very low blood glucose levels if they don't eat regularly – a condition called reactive hypoglycaemia – so it's worth 'dipping your toe' into fasting slowly to see how your body reacts. Visit the www.fastdiet.co.uk website for a list of those who should take additional care or avoid fasting diets for a significant period of time.

How insulin can contribute to weight gain

Every time we eat, we produce the hormone insulin. Insulin is a storage hormone – its job is to facilitate movement of glucose out of the blood stream into cells, and promote storage as glycogen in the liver and muscles. It also reduces lipolysis (the breakdown of fat) so that glucose is preferentially used up as fuel, which is obviously not good news if you want to use up and reduce body fat! Insulin also stimulates the conversion of any excess glucose into fat, so not only is it reducing the amount of fat you are using up, it is increasing the amount you are storing. As insulin secretion is most strongly stimulated by eating carbohydrate foods, this illustrates the connection between eating too much sugar or refined carbohydrates with a high glycaemic index (fast absorption rate), and weight gain. With the current epidemic of obesity and diabetes, it is now considered that we should eat less frequently rather than graze through the day, to limit insulin secretion. Research on the effects of increased insulin secretion is partly what has fuelled the current plethora of low carb, high protein, high fat and fasting diets seen today.

'Consume only what your body needs, when it needs it.'

Maintaining weight loss

Once you have reached your target weight through intermittent fasting, you may be able to maintain your new weight by fasting for just one day a week, although your calorie requirements (BMR) will be reduced at your new lower weight, so as soon as you regularly consume more calories than you are using up, you will begin to regain weight. The best ways to maintain a healthy weight are:

- Have lower calorie days as required, going back to the 5:2 regime if needed, or even 4:3 to undo a short period of overindulgence

- Use exercise to use up more calories, with the added benefits of improving blood glucose control and insulin sensitivity, and creating more lean muscle that will increase your metabolic rate.

The Paleo diet

Paleolithic diets are based upon eating a Stone Age diet, first promoted by Dr. Walter L Voegtlin in 1975. Since then, variations on the original Stone Age diet have occurred, such as the Caveman diet, the Hunter-gatherer diet and the Paleo diet. The human body adapts very slowly to changes in the way that we eat, so as the Paleolithic era was pre-agricultural, foods that would not have been available during that time are excluded from the diet, as it is thought our digestive system may struggle to digest foods such as those listed below:

- Cereals such as wheat, barley, rye, and oats

- Refined sugar

- Potatoes

- Processed foods

- Legumes (peas, peanuts, soya)

- Dairy

- Refined vegetable oils

- Root vegetables.

There are several different 'stone age' diets, and some formats of this type of diet allow low-fat dairy products and root vegetables to be included. All versions of the diet are based upon lean proteins (meat from grass fed animals), fish, eggs, fruit, vegetables, nuts, seeds, natural oils and naturally occurring sugars such as honey. The Paleo diet is a form of 'clean eating', excluding or limiting processed, refined foods. With the exclusion of starchy carbohydrates (potatoes, bread, pasta, rice and cereals), this way of eating can be a low carbohydrate diet, although there is no limit to the amount of carbohydrates you can eat, and raw honey, coconut nectar and pure maple syrup, are all allowed.

As long as you haven't got a sweet tooth and consume lots of allowed sugars, the diet may be relatively low in carbohydrates but rich in lean protein and plant foods, which contribute all-important fibre, vitamins, minerals and phyto-chemicals. The elimination of such a wide range of foods like grains, dairy and processed foods means this way of eating is more than likely to lead to some weight loss. Some studies report positive health outcomes from consuming a Paleo diet, including weight loss, improved blood sugar control and a reduction in the risk factors for heart disease.

Ketogenic diets

A diet that is high in fat and low in carbohydrates is a ketogenic diet. The Atkins Diet was a low-carbohydrate, high fat weight loss regime in the 1970-80s, but at the time it was heavily criticized by health professionals, much as ketogenic diets are condemned now. However, there is increasing evidence that suggests that the ketogenic diet is an effective way to lose weight, and also improves blood glucose control and heart health.

A standard ketogenic diet is typically 70 – 75% (or unrestricted) fat, 20% protein (40 – 60g daily) and 5 – 10% carbohydrate (usually no more than 30g daily, although everyone goes 'into' ketosis on differing carbohydrate intakes). Whereas 58% of proteins are glucogenic and can be turned into glucose, only 10% of the fat molecule (glylcerol) can be used for gluconeogenesis (making glucose), so a high fat diet is much more ketonic than a high protein diet. Ketones are said to be an efficient source of energy for many organs in the body, although their acidity does require constant buffering to enable the blood to maintain a healthy pH. The low carbohydrate intake forces the body to obtain energy from fat instead of glucose or stored glycogen. However, during very low carbohydrate intake or starvation, fat (which has been converted into Acetyl Co-enzyme A), cannot enter the citric acid cycle to be fully broken down, so it produces substances called ketones.

As carbohydrates are so restricted, fibre is also extremely low, so it is important to include as many non-starchy vegetables in the diet as possible, as these are low in carbohydrate content but high in fibre and water. Side effects of ketosis can include constipation, lack of energy, brain 'fog', dizziness, insomnia and cravings, although it is said these symptoms disappear once the body has adapted to being in ketosis. The breath can smell fruity as acetone (a ketone which isn't used in the body) is eliminated mainly via respiration in the lungs.

Those following the earlier Atkins diet typically consumed mostly animal protein foods such as meat, dairy and eggs, so the type of fat eaten was predominantly saturated. Although more recent evidence suggests that saturated fat may not carry the health warnings originally thought, there are some moderations of the classic ketogenic diet that include more unsaturated fats, whereas the classic ketogenic diet does not discern between the types of fat consumed.

How do ketogenic diets reduce bodyweight?

Ketosis metabolism in the body has a high energy consumption, so it has been proposed that this is what induces weight loss, although no change in resting metabolic rate is found on a ketogenic diet. Gluconeogenesis (producing glucose from non-carbohydrate sources) can use up approximately 400–600 calories daily. There is substantial evidence of higher satiety from consuming protein and fatty foods, and also effects upon appetite control hormones such as ghrelin and leptin.

A study by Saslow et al. (2014) found that a lower calorie diet did not present better weight loss when compared with a ketogenic diet, and carbohydrate restriction made it easier to adhere to low energy intake long-term than restricting fat intake. Greater weight loss was achieved on the ketogenic diet, along with improved glycaemic (blood glucose) control. A meta-analysis of studies (Gibson et al, 2015) showed that individuals were less hungry and exhibited greater fullness/satiety on very low calorie diets; those following a ketogenic low calorie diet were also less hungry and had a reduced desire to eat. These appetite adaptations occurred during energy restriction, which is known to usually increase appetite in obese people, so the satiating effects of a ketogenic or fasting diet may be instrumental in longevity of a weight reducing eating plan. So the likely mechanisms via which weight loss is achieved on a higher protein and/or ketogenic (high fat) diet are:

- Thermic effect of more protein in the diet
- Improved appetite control through higher satiety effect of proteins

- Reduction in appetite due to effects on appetite control hormones such as ghrelin
- Possible direct appetite suppressant action of the ketone bodies
- Reduction in lipogenesis (fat formation) and increased lipolysis (fat breakdown)
- Greater metabolic efficiency (more energy used up with ketogenic metabolism)
- Increased metabolic costs of gluconeogenesis.

Drawbacks of a ketogenic diet

A ketogenic diet is an extreme diet, and not for everyone. There is a risk of developing constipation, and some experts express concerns over long-term micronutrient deficiencies and the risk of conditions such as osteoporosis if the diet is not nutritionally balanced. In extreme starvation, the level of ketones could create acidosis, and some experts say there is also a greater risk of Type 1 diabetics going into a state known as ketoacidosis, although this is different to ketosis, and only occurs if they have consumed too many carbohydrates (which would mean they weren't really following a ketogenic diet) and not taken on board enough insulin.

Ketosis is when the body is using fat as its main fuel and producing ketones, which occurs with a very low carbohydrate intake, on a ketogenic or fasting diet. It is sometimes referred to as 'nutritional ketosis'. Diabetic ketoacidosis is a dangerous and potentially fatal condition that mostly occurs during 'starvation' in people with Type 1 diabetes, when not enough insulin has been administered. Glucose cannot enter the cells without insulin, so the body breaks down fat and protein into ketones at an alarming rate, far above what is seen in ketosis. Ketoacidosis develops when there are both high ketone levels and high blood glucose.

A ketogenic diet is not recommended if you have pancreatic issues, pyruvate carboxylase deficiency, porphyria or are trying for a baby, pregnant or breastfeeding, and it is recommended that those with any type of diabetes work with a qualified health professional if considering a ketogenic diet.

Paleo-Keto diet

It is possible to combine elements of paleo eating with a ketogenic diet to create what may be perceived as a healthier ketogenic diet. Fat intake would still have to be high enough to enter ketosis, although the types of fats consumed would be from fish, shellfish and grass fed animals rather than processed meats, and if sticking with the non-dairy rule of paleo eating, there would be no dairy foods. However, some paleo diets allow butter made from grass fed animals. Any sweeteners used would have to be non-nutritive (no calories) 'natural' sweeteners to comply with the 'clean eating' element of paleo diets, although from a nutritional health point of view, no sweeteners are recommended.

The MCT (Medium chain triglyceride) diet – can coconuts help weight loss?

The MCT diet is based upon a standard ketogenic diet but includes mostly medium chain fatty acids as the type of fat eaten. This diet also allows a higher consumption of protein and carbohydrates due to the fact that medium chain triglycerides yield more ketones per unit of dietary energy than other types of fat. Coconut oil is a rich source of medium chain triglycerides (and other types of fatty acids), although it is not always used in MCT diets and trials.

One trial reporting results on 31 subjects showed that consumption of MCT oil (8 – 12 carbons long) as part of a weight-loss plan improved weight loss compared with olive oil (which contains high levels of longer chain oleic oil, 18 carbons long). The difference in weight loss over 16 weeks was 1.67kg on average, and total fat mass and intra-abdominal adipose tissue were both lower with MCT consumption than with olive oil consumption. In other trials, increased shunting of dietary fat towards oxidation resulting in diminished fat storage, and enhanced exercise endurance have both been reported following MCT intake. However, no significant differences in changes in weight, BMI or central adiposity were found in a study by Khaw et al (2018), who compared the effects of consuming 50g coconut oil in comparison to 50g olive oil or butter on blood lipid profile, weight, fat distribution and metabolic markers.

Mumme and Stonehouse (2015) reviewed studies that had compared the effects of MCTs to long-chain triglycerides on weight loss and body composition. Compared with longer chain fats, MCTs decreased body weight by 0.51kg more, waist circumference by 1.46cm more, hip circumference by 0.79cm more, total body fat reduced by 0.39kg more, total subcutaneous fat 0.46kg more and visceral fat reduced by 0.55kg more. Their conclusion was that MCTs in the diet could potentially induce modest reductions in body weight and composition. The simple chemistry of this is that a medium chain triglyceride (or medium chain fatty acid) is not as long as a longer chain fatty acid, so there are fewer bonds and less available energy. For this reason, it is suggested that medium chain triglycerides provide only 8.3 kcals per gram, as opposed to the 9 kcals per gram that fats are generally said to contain.

But before you go out and start eating coconuts every day, note that they actually only contain around 13 – 15% medium chain triglycerides! However, eating coconuts and pure coconut oil is a more natural way to consume medium chain triglycerides than using MCT oils, which are often a processed oil containing MCTs, and may not contain any coconut at all.

Fat consumption is a highly debated subject. Current UK guidelines advise that no more than 35% of energy intake should come from fat, and that saturated fat should be limited. However, the PURE study reported that total fat and even saturated fat were not associated with cardiovascular disease, and instead, a correlation between higher carbohydrate intake and higher risk of total mortality was found (Dehghan et al., 2017).

Pros and cons of low carbohydrate diets

Both higher protein (Paleo) type diets and high fat (ketogenic) diets have low carbohydrate content. All meat/fish products including processed foods such as cured, smoked and tinned meats are included in the classic ketogenic diet, but the Paleo diet doesn't promote salty, processed meats. Paleo eating includes more fruit and vegetables than ketogenic diets, providing essential fibre, and a wider range of vitamins and minerals. The Paleo diet also promotes more natural fats from pasture-fed livestock, fish and seafood as well as nuts, seeds and their oils, rather than all types of fat included in the ketogenic diet. Although more recent research has indicated that cardiovascular health issues linked to eating too much saturated fat may not be evident, there is still a plethora of research promoting the benefits of unsaturated fats over saturated fats, so the Paleo way of eating appears to be a healthier choice in this respect.

What both diets have in common is that carbohydrate intake is reduced (particularly in ketogenic diets). Obese individuals often have insulin resistance, which means that dietary carbohydrate cannot be metabolized properly and more of it is converted into fat, so low fat, relatively high carbohydrate diets such as those promoted for weight loss over the past twenty years have only contributed to the current obesity crisis. The potential benefits of following reduced carbohydrate, higher protein or higher fat diets for weight loss have been shown to also have beneficial effects upon glucose management and insulin resistance. Research also indicates that the ketogenic diet may show better overall results than the low-fat, moderate carbohydrate diet that is currently favoured by the NHS.

There are many documented health benefits from consuming whole-grains, beans, legumes and starchy vegetables, such as decreased risk of bowel cancer, reduced cholesterol, lower incidence of heart disease, and better blood glucose control, and all of these foods also supply B vitamins and a range of minerals. However, studies have also shown that cholesterol and the risk of heart disease are reduced with low carbohydrate intake, and glucose control is also improved on a low carbohydrate diet. So it seems that if plenty of vegetables are included in a high protein or high fat diet, these will provide the benefits listed below and make Paleo and ketogenic diets a healthier option.

- Fibre for a healthy bowel and for good cholesterol management

- Vitamins, minerals and phytonutrients for general good health

- Vegetables are still low in carbohydrate (starch) content, so including this food group will not overly increase overall carbohydrate or calorie intake

- Most vegetables have a low glycaemic index (GI) so will not elevate blood glucose levels and incite high insulin release

- Including vegetables also provides greater dietary diversity and a wider range of food options, improving the longevity of any diet.

Fruit may also convey many of these benefits but contains more sugars, so lower levels are likely to be included in any type of low carbohydrate diet. Another criticism of the Paleo and some ketogenic diets is that excluding dairy foods limits calcium intake. Including nuts, seeds and dark green leafy vegetables in an eating regime provides some calcium, and fish containing small bones is also an excellent source. Even if calcium-containing beans and pulses are excluded, with careful inclusion of other calcium-rich foods, sufficient calcium can be consumed without dairy in the diet. However, when embarking upon a long-term diet that excludes any food group, consulting with a nutritional therapist, nutritionist or dietician would ensure that the diet contains not just sufficient calcium, but all the nutrients required for continued good health.

Summing Up

Different diets will always come and go. This chapter has reviewed the most current popular diets. Whilst there is clearly evidence that fasting, higher protein/reduced carbohydrate and ketogenic diets can reduce body weight, it is important to base a healthy long term diet upon the most rigorous research and the best elements of nutrition.

- Intermittent fasting appears to provide a way of reducing caloric intake without reducing metabolic rate

- Fasting can help you to lose weight and body fat

- Ketogenic diets can create weight loss and have been shown to be more successful than low calorie diets in some research

- Reducing sugars and carbohydrates appears to be a healthy way to reduce calorie intake and lose weight, whilst simultaneously improving glycaemic (glucose) and insulin metabolism

- Paleo diets can provide a healthy way of 'eating clean', although sugar intake should still be limited

- Although some research shows that medium chain triglycerides may enhance weight loss, differences between these and other fats are minimal. However, including natural coconut as part of your diet imparts some health benefits.

9

Weight Loss for Life

How many times have you successfully lost weight but failed to keep it off? Slimming clubs are full of people who have repeatedly yo-yoed between weight loss and weight gain, and 'fat and thin wardrobes'. Losing weight is one thing, but keeping it off is another. Every dieter wants to stop 'dieting' and create a lifestyle that will enable them to maintain a healthy weight for life. So let's take a look at what long-term weight maintenance involves.

A long term eating plan that will enable you to keep your weight within 7lbs of your target weight has to be three things:

1 It has to be enjoyable otherwise you won't stick to it

2 It has to match your calorie intake with the amount of energy (calories) you are using up to provide weight maintenance

3 It has to provide all the nutrients required for good health.

Balancing calories for life

Although this may sound onerous, this doesn't necessarily mean weighing food portions and counting calories, it simply means that you need to keep an eye on your overall calorie intake and expenditure – the big picture rather than individual meals.

What is a healthy diet?

A healthy diet should contain all the nutrients that are essential for good health with a wide range of foods in balanced proportions, providing adequate caloric intake to maintain a healthy body weight. A diet for life should tick all of these boxes:

- At least five portions of vegetables are eaten daily (with some fruit)
- Protein foods such as meat, fish, eggs or soya are eaten two to three times daily
- Sugar and refined carbohydrates should be strictly limited
- Food contains an adequate amount of vitamins and minerals
- A wide variety of food is eaten
- At least two litres of water are consumed daily
- Processed foods are kept to a minimum.

'If you cannot follow a diet plan for life, it is not going to provide you with long term weight maintenance.'

Your choice of simply balancing your calorie intake with expenditure, following a low carbohydrate diet with either more protein (paleo) or fat (keto), or trying intermittent fasting will determine the proportions of carbohydrates, protein and fat in your diet. Considering all the scientific evidence available, it is recommended that your diet should contain no more than 50% carbohydrate (and ideally less than this), and most of this should come from vegetables, nuts, seeds and fruit. The remainder of the diet provides protein and fat-rich fish, eggs, meat, natural fats and vegetable oils. Depending upon your chosen eating plan, some dairy and vegetable proteins such as beans, pulses or soya may also be consumed.

Eating a wide variety of foods and choosing whole foods over processed foods will help to ensure that your diet still contains vital vitamins and minerals. Checking which nutrients are in any food/food group you may have reduced, and seeking these nutrients in alternative foods or supplements, will help to address potential long-term deficiencies.

Going on a diet versus adapting your own eating regime

Changing to a very different eating regime or diet can be very difficult, which is why many new diets fall by the wayside after a number of days or weeks. When you come off of a diet, you return to your usual eating practices (the habits that created the weight gain in the first place), and gradually regain all the weight you lost. So, it follows that a successful diet must begin with adjusting your usual eating habits until you have a normal, healthy eating pattern that balances your calorie intake with your calorie expenditure. This balance should include making full use of the metabolic advantages that eating a little more protein or fat, and less carbohydrate, provides.

Getting through the year – a guide to get you over those hurdles!

There will always be a number of times throughout the year when a higher calorie intake is likely, or when your usual diet is put on hold. These may be occasions involving one large meal (birthdays, anniversaries, celebrations), or times of the year when calorie-dodging is more difficult for a longer period of time (Christmas, holidays). You may also experience changes in your life that have a significant effect upon your food choices, such as a change in job, a change in home life, or a new partner. All of these things come to test us, and so you must be ready to meet and survive these challenges.

Whilst occasions such as Christmas or a holiday are likely to change your normal healthy eating routine, the trick is to avoid letting these events take over your entire diet for longer than necessary. Within every long term healthy eating plan there will occasionally be more sumptuous meals, treats and days with high calorie intakes – and this is fine – within limitation. Consider the bigger picture, the weekly energy balance rather than the daily intake, and plan how to offset those higher calorie meals or days against lower energy consumption. We know these events are coming every year, so we really have no excuse to be unprepared and unable to cope with these occasions. A little 'damage limitation' is all that is required.

Of course, you could simply just exercise more to balance your higher calorie intake with greater energy expenditure. However, at these times, exercise habits are often also likely to change – usually not for the better! So here are some tips to help you get through the year(s) and weigh in at the same weight (or maybe even lower) at the end of the year.

Annual damage limitation plan

New Year

First of all, deal with the extras from the Yuletide season to put an end to over-indulgence!

- Give away or even throw away left over chocolates. You're probably down to the strawberry creams and Turkish delights anyway, so take a deep breath and clear away the temptation.

- Deep freeze left over mince pies so you have to defrost them one at a time to eat them – a mince pie sitting in the kitchen is a mince pie waiting to be eaten!

- Christmas cake is another temptation (if you must have one in the first place) – if you can't freeze leftovers, throw it out with unwanted mince pies for the birds.

- Launch yourself into some new year's resolutions and take up a new activity to use up additional calories.

- Try a healthy detox to give you a kick-start to the year.

Valentines Day and Easter

These two events have chocolate in common – if you are not on a strict eating regime that doesn't include chocolate, and just can't stop at one, try these tips to get you past this chocoholic disaster area.

- Tell well-meaning family and friends not to buy you chocolate – and mean it!

- If it's a well-loved tradition for someone to buy you chocolate for Valentines Day or Easter, ask for dark chocolate instead. It contains more nutrients and less sugar, and the richer taste can make it less likely to be guzzled as quickly.

- Opt for lower calorie options such as unfilled or smaller eggs.

- Arrange to do something different instead – plan a spa day for two or an activity day for the family.

Spring

Spring is a great time to try a detox, fill up on healthy spring vegetables such as asparagus, broccoli and spring cabbage, and give your lifestyle a spring clean! With warmer temperatures and lighter nights it becomes easier to exercise outside and we're also more likely to drink more water. Why not set yourself a few goals to achieve, such as drinking 2 litres of water a day, completing so many exercise minutes weekly, or making sure you eat five servings of fruit and vegetables daily? Eating a healthy diet should be about increasing the range of foods you eat, not limiting it.

Summer and healthy BBQs

Summer is a time of barbeques and holidays... which could be a dieter's dream or a weight loss nightmare... you just need to indulge in the right types of foods.

If your idea of a BBQ conjures up images of burgers and sausages covered in your sauce of choice and sandwiched in a floury white bun, you need a BBQ makeover! Alfresco eating is only good for us if the food is healthy – include these healthy foods in your BBQs and alfresco dining for tasty and healthy meals.

Sweet potatoes are exactly that – sweeter and less starchy than normal potatoes. They're packed with anti-oxidant and super-nutrient beta-carotene (the best natural nutrient we have to help counteract the effects of sun damage to the skin). Bake on the BBQ as you would a normal spud.

Sweet corn is another vegetable packed with beta-carotene, which acts as an important anti-oxidant and converts into Vitamin A as required for healthy eyes, skin and immune function. Wrap each corn cob in foil with some chopped garlic and chili to give a fantastic smell and taste whilst adding even more nutrients.

Choose from spinach, watercress or rocket – all three are packed with magnesium, potassium, iron, calcium and Vitamin C. You could rub the tomatoes with olive oil and roast them with garlic beforehand for a real Mediterranean taste. Mix the leaves with the tomatoes and cubes of ripe avocado. Although not shy on the calorie count and therefore excluded in many diets, avocados are packed with goodness – they contain lutein, a type of anti-oxidant carotenoid known for promoting good eye health, and monounsaturated (healthy) fats. Add a tablespoon of pine nuts for a little crunch and more nutrients, and a splash of balsamic vinegar if desired.

Sliced green/red/orange/yellow peppers, onions, mushrooms, courgettes, baby corn on the cob... try and create a rainbow of healthy colour on your vegetable skewers. A kebab like this provides a wealth of nutritious and tasty foods.

The perfect food to include in your BBQ to get your intake of omega 3 fatty acids – definitely a healthier option than the usual BBQ burger! Just place salmon fillets in foil parcels and add to the BBQ for the last 10 minutes or so. Any type of fish can be eaten instead.

Holidays

A holiday is likely to be the longest period of time that you are out of your normal routine, so it's no surprise that many people come back from a fortnight in the sun carrying an extra pound in weight for every day they've been away! But your yearly 'mini-sabbatical' need not undo all that 'hard work' you've put in over the preceding months to fit into your bikini or swimming trunks. You want to return home looking and feeling even better than when you arrived, not like you need a detox week at a health spa.

There is really no reason for you to change your eating habits whilst you are on holiday, and the good news is that all those tools you have developed which have enabled you to lose weight can be put to even better use in a holiday situation.

Toolbox of holiday help

'Tomatoes contain a fantastic phytonutrient called lycopene, which has been linked with reduced incidence of breast and prostate cancer.'

- Don't go overboard! You have plenty of time to enjoy an ice cream, an alcoholic tipple or a dessert, so don't feel that you have to over-indulge in everything all at once – particularly if you are staying in an all-inclusive resort.

- All-inclusive holidays can make it difficult to employ calorie limitation and portion control, so when you're booking a holiday, consider this. You may be more likely to eat healthily when choosing from a menu, rather than filling your plate as full as you like.

- Drink water through the day to hydrate you and help you avoid sugary and higher calorie drinks such as alcohol, juices, fizzy drinks and holiday cocktails. The water will also ensure that you don't feel thirsty, which can be misinterpreted as hunger and prompt snacking.

- Being dehydrated can result in drinking more alcoholic beverages – and taking in more calories. Stay well hydrated with water, and then you can sip at your alcoholic drinks and engage in damage limitation!

- Choose foods you might not usually eat, such as different types of fish, shellfish or vegetables – eating healthily can be easier on holiday when someone else has prepared a range of foods for you.

- Pass on the breadbasket. It's not just the bread, which is usually an unnecessary addition to a meal, but the spread you put on it. Adding this to your daily intake over a couple of weeks will make a difference to your post-holiday weight, and might even reawaken some bad habits.

- If food is served buffet-style, remember the golden rules about portion control:

    Choose a smaller plate

    Eat slowly

    Have smaller amounts of things that you want to try rather than full portions of everything

    Fill up your plate with lower calorie vegetables – the volume of food that we eat affects our food intake in subsequent courses and later in the day

    Don't eat food just because it's available – if there is nothing you want to eat for dessert, don't have anything.

Offset additional calorie intake with activity

You're more likely to have spare time whilst you're on holiday, so try to keep off the sun lounger and stay active:

- Walk or swim every day; create a healthy habit of swimming a set number of lengths in the pool or taking a long walk before or after dinner

- Take long walks on the beach or around wherever you are staying

- Try a new activity – wind surfing, kayaking, scuba diving, snorkeling, cycling...

- Stay active on the beach with a Frisbee or ball game

- Use the hotel facilities: gym, table tennis, tennis, crazy golf, organized walks...

Picnics and days out

A day out needn't upset your healthy eating or weight maintenance. Just choose healthy options and try and include some activity to counteract any additional energy intake.

Healthy picnic options

- Take plenty of water with you to drink throughout the day.

- Take a healthy fruit salad if you must have dessert – mixed berries, kiwi, melon, mango, red grapes and cherries...

- Instead of crisps take raw vegetables such as baby corn, mange tout, baby tomatoes, carrots, asparagus, celery and cucumber sticks.

- Avoid packing pastry based foods such as pork pies and quiches, or shop bought scotch eggs and pies, all laden with refined fats, starches and salt. Instead, take a home made frittata and salad, olives, boiled eggs, lean meats or cooked fish.

Working off that picnic!

- Instead of going to the park or beach and sitting down to picnic all day, make the picnic part of a walk. You can buy rucksacks that come complete with plates, plastic glasses, napkins and cutlery (don't worry; there's space for food too). Instead of driving to your picnic spot, plan a walk from your house, carry your lunch with you and enjoy a picnic lunch en route.

- Picnic games. If you're loading up the car with blankets, deckchairs, and a portable stove, you can certainly find space for a ball and bats. A beach ball or football, or cricket ball and stumps provides a perfect opportunity for some pre- and post-picnic games. Really stuck for space? The Frisbee leaves you with no excuses!

- Why not picnic somewhere that you can take part in an activity? Many popular picnic sites are close to water – try boating, kayaking or other water sports, or even take a dip if it's safe. Work up an appetite!

- Why not cycle to your picnic? You could plan a full day's route, and the picnic can be carried in a bicycle basket or in a rucksack. Having to cycle back should also help you to limit any alcoholic beverages you might have consumed.

Autumn

As the weather cools and nights draw in, we naturally find ourselves wanting warm, sometimes stodgy food. After a summer of salads, this can seem like a difficult time for calorie control and weight maintenance, but just remember that if a food has a higher calorie density (for instance, compare potatoes with broccoli), just have less of it. Autumn is a great time for all root vegetables, but choosing those with a higher water and fibre content will help you to keep calories in check. Check out this table to compare the carbohydrate, fibre and water content and calorie count per 100g of uncooked autumn vegetables.

Vegetable	Fibre	Carbohydrate	Water	Calories
Potato	1.2	17	80.3	72
Parsnip	4.7	12.9	78.7	66
Carrot	2.5	4.9	90.5	24
Pumpkin	1.1	2.1	94.9	13
Turnip	1.9	2.0	93.1	12

Source of information: McCance and Widdowson's 'The Composition of Foods. 6th ed. 2002'.

Weight maintenance in Autumn

- Make your own soups – this way you know exactly what has gone in to the soup and there are no creams or starches increasing calorie count. Begin with leeks or onions and garlic, and then base your soups on seasonal vegetables such as pumpkin, squash, carrot or parsnip.

- Stew apples or pears for a healthy breakfast, dessert or supper option. Top with cinnamon and a sprinkle of nuts or seeds.

Winter

Continue with all the good habits you have created through autumn, and put those tasty root vegetables to even more use by swapping the starch-rich potatoes for lower calorie alternatives:

- Mash carrots, turnips and parsnips instead of mashed potatoes

- Instead of boiled or mashed potatoes AND roasted potatoes, just opt for roasted parsnips and carrots

- Add swede and celeriac to stews and soups instead of potato.

Winter holidays

Employ all the tips from the summer holiday section if you are staying in a hotel or eating out, and make the most of any activities available to offset any additional (and likely) calorie intake – ski-ing, snowboarding, walking, trekking...

Christmas

Along with holidays, this is probably the most likely time of the year that you may gain weight, so it's worth creating a damage limitation plan that will enable you to get to January without having to spend half of next year losing the weight you've gained in December.

In the run up to Christmas...

'Christmas Day is just one day... why eat differently for a whole month?!'

- Plan healthy eating days before and after each Christmas party to balance the higher calorie intake. Counteract the copious calorie intake with lots of water, vegetables and healthy protein foods – your body will thank you for the mini-detox and you'll still be able to fit into that little black dress or tuxedo on New Year's Eve.

- Engage in intermittent fasting before, during and after Christmas to help balance out overall calorie intake.

- Don't let your exercise slip! Try to keep your workouts going right through Christmas – even try to increase it to counteract the additional calories you're likely to eat.

- A few careful choices at the Christmas parties and buffets will prevent you gaining a couple of extra pounds:

    Choose raw vegetable crudités instead of bread sticks or deep fried dippers

    Opt for plain fish or meat rather than pastry snacks

    Eat before you go out to prevent overindulging at the buffet table

    Choose white wine spritzers rather than a glass of wine, or alternate alcoholic drinks with sparkling water to halve those calories.

Yuletide tips for Christmas day!

- Christmas dinner is typically a large plateful of food – have a little bit of everything, but keep the overall meal portion size within reason

- Do you really want three types of potatoes and bread sauce? Limit the starchy carbohydrates by only having your favorite

- Use all the usual tips to help you avoid overeating – eat slowly, sip between mouthfuls, and stop when you feel full

- Alternate alcoholic drinks through the day with some sparkling water to reduce calorie intake, or only indulge with meals

- Don't put chocolates, nuts and snacks out – you'll only pick at them all day

- Save Christmas pudding until later – it reduces your lunchtime food intake and will replace mince pies or chocolates later on in the evening

- Have a smaller portion of Christmas pudding, and top it with Greek yoghurt or crème fraîche instead of cream

- Visit **www.weightlossresources.co.uk** for lower calorie food ideas over the Christmas period.

If you are given any high calorie Christmas presents before Christmas day, consider wrapping them up for other people rather than consuming them yourself.

Keeping an eye on your weight

How many times have you heard or said 'the weight just seems to creep on'? But body fat doesn't accumulate on our hips or stomachs overnight... we put it there with hours of hard work, munching our way through too much food and glugging our way through alcohol or sugary drinks... and then not doing enough exercise to work it all off. If only we'd kept an eye on our weight, and noticed when we gained an inch, or a few pounds, it would have been so much easier and quicker to get back to where we were!

So this is an important part of your life-long weight maintenance plan... keep your eye on things. Set yourself a range based upon weight, dress size or measurements that you know you will realistically vary within over a typical month, and maybe just check this measurement once monthly. Once you begin to gain more than 4lbs, or one inch, or an additional dress size over your maintenance weight, do something about it immediately.

Remember, there are approximately 3500 calories in a pound of stored body fat, so if you have gained 4 pounds in fat, you already have to find ways to create a calorie deficit of approximately 14,000 calories (it will be less than this as some energy is used up just metabolizing the excess fat for energy). It already sounds monumental, so it's no wonder it can take many months to reduce body weight by a couple of stones.

Ways to get back on track

- Limit your intake of alcohol, biscuits, cakes, chocolate, ice cream, sauces, fatty meats, sausages and pastry based foods

- If you have stopped measuring or limiting starchy foods such as cereals, rice, pasta, bread and potatoes, measure and limit your intake of these calorie dense foods, or even better, cut them out

- Go back to the things you did to reduce your body weight initially, and re-introduce some of your successful healthy habits

- Keep an eye on portion sizes – it may not be what you're eating, but how much

- Snack on raw vegetables if you must eat between meals, and make sure you haven't slipped into unhealthy snacking habits such as eating biscuits, cakes or high calorie dips

- Consider some intermittent fasting days to help with weight loss

- Increase your exercise – and if you are already doing a lot of exercise, or have no time to do more, increase the intensity level instead.

Increasing exercise intensity

You may find yourself in a situation where you are eating a healthy, calorie controlled, portion-controlled diet and exercising regularly, but you are still gaining or unable to lose weight. In this situation many people make the mistake of reducing their calorie intake too low, which may lower metabolic rate and reduce the amount of calories the body can utilise. This is counterproductive to weight loss.

The thing to do in this situation is to find ways of using up more energy (calories) rather than further reducing your calorie intake. The body becomes very accustomed to whatever activities it regularly undertakes and expends fewer calories as it adapts to the activity being done. To counteract this, you will need to find ways of raising the exercise intensity so that you can increase your calorie expenditure once again.

Here are some ways to increase exercise intensity and calorie expenditure:

- Do some higher intensity training sessions such as HIIT
- Exercise for longer or add additional sessions into your week
- Do an exercise routine (for example in the gym) back to front
- Increase the resistance or speed on the rower, cycle, step trainer or treadmill
- Change the programme on the rower, cycle, step trainer or treadmill
- Change your normal walking or running route
- Walk the same route but carry a rucksack containing water bottles or other weights
- Get a new gym routine
- Go to a new fitness class
- Take up a new activity
- Reduce your rest time when you exercise – less rest between lengths in the pool, less time between machines or sets in the gym, put more effort in during your exercise class
- Introduce interval training (spurts of higher intensity exercise) into your normal routine, or adapt your existing interval training to increase intensity further.

Don't forget, you're in this for the long haul, so consider the bigger picture... one biscuit is not a problem, a 'blow out' weekend won't undo everything, but you have to offset each indulgence with a bit of extra exercise or an extra healthy day. Just keep it all in balance.

Nobody wants to be 'on a diet' their entire life, but balancing your calorie intake need not entail constantly denying yourself the foods you want to eat. In creating a healthy diet and lifestyle that you can maintain for life, you are stepping away from restrictive, short term fad diets and the subsequent boomerang of weight regain. Long-term weight maintenance is a credit-debit arrangement in which you must balance your calorie intake with your energy expenditure. That may mean offsetting indulgences with healthier eating, and exercising to help keep everything in balance, but doing this will mean that you can have your cake – and eat it – every now and then!

Summing Up

So now you have the low-down on the most popular and effective weight loss diets, have noted your portion sizes and dusted off your exercise goals, here is a quick summary of the best weight loss options available to you.

Simply reduce calorie intake and/or increase expenditure

Using the basic energy balance equation, if you cut out processed, sugary foods and snacks (which will also improve insulin metabolism), you will have a healthier diet and a lower calorie intake, and are likely to lose weight. Throwing in some additional exercise will increase the weight loss and health benefits. You can follow the 80-20 rule with this weight loss regime: eat healthily 80% of the time, and for 20% of meals, allow yourself foods/drinks that you really enjoy but know you can't consume regularly and still lose/maintain weight loss if you consumed them all the time. Fasting – particularly intermittent fasting – is another way to reduce your calorie intake.

Portion control

It may be that your diet is healthy but you simply eat too much. Reducing portions will also benefit glycaemic and insulin control as well as induce weight loss, and although it can be psychologically tricky to change the amount you eat, there are lots of tips to help you in Chapter 6.

Reducing carbohydrates and increasing protein and/or fat

Consuming fewer carbohydrates – especially sugars and refined starches – is beneficial for glycaemic control and insulin metabolism; it will aid weight loss and provide health benefits. Eating more protein can help you sustain a lower food intake through increased satiety, and also provide a metabolic advantage as your body is using up more energy metabolizing protein. Although healthy fats found in vegetable oils, olives, avocado, nuts and seeds should form a part of your diet, eating more fatty foods is only beneficial for weight loss if you are in ketosis. If you eat more fats whilst still consuming a moderate amount of carbohydrates you will still be producing amounts of insulin that will help to store the fat rather than use it for energy. All you will have succeeded in doing is eating more calories!

So remember…

- Only a healthy, balanced diet can create life long weight maintenance
- Make use of the metabolic advantage that eating less carbohydrate and a little more protein can give you
- Consider the bigger picture and balance out indulgences with healthier options
- Aim to use the 80-20 rule if you need a little dietary indulgence
- Balance overall energy input with energy expenditure
- Plan your way through high risk times such as holidays and Christmas
- Keep an eye on your weight and start to act as soon as you go over your normal weight range.

'Eat to live, rather than live to eat!'

Help List

Online weight loss resources

BMI and waist: hip ratio calculator website
http://www.bmi-calculator.net/waist-to-hip-ratio-calculator/waist-circumference.php

Slimming world in the UK and Republic of Ireland
https://www.slimmingworld.co.uk

Weight watchers in the UK and Republic of Ireland
https://www.weightwatchers.com/uk/
www.weightwatchers.ie
All weight loss groups provide recipes, menus, information, weight loss and activity challenges and on-line group communities.

Intermittent fasting – websites of the popularized fast diet and 5:2 eating plan
www.thefastdiet.co.uk
https://the5-2dietbook.com/books

Diet Doctor
This is a comprehensive website sharing information on fasting, low carb and keto diets.
https://www.dietdoctor.com

Weight Loss Resources
Weight Loss Resources Ltd, 29 Metro Centre, Woodston, Peterborough, PE2 7UH
Tel: 01733 345592
helpteam@weightlossresources.co.uk
https://www.weightlossresources.co.uk
This website is an extensive resource of calorie and nutritional information. It also provides weight loss tools such as a BMI calculator, a user friendly on line food diary and exercise log (with calorie intake and expenditure calculated for you), a wide range of credible nutrition information, tips and recipes. You can plot your progress on a weight loss chart, post questions and communicate with their online weight loss community.

NHS

An extensive range of dietary and exercise tools to help you lose weight.
https://www.nhs.uk/Livewell/weight-loss-guide/Pages/losing-weight-getting-started.aspx
https://www.nhs.uk/livewell/healthy-eating/Pages/Healthyeating.aspx
This website provides information on national healthy eating initiatives such as '5 A DAY' and 'Change4Life', as well as providing nutrition and diet information for the general public.

Weight Wise – British Dietetic Association

www.bdaweightwise.com
This is a website run by the British Dietetic Association which offers a wealth of free weight loss tools and credible dietary advice. You can post questions, calculate your ideal weight, and print off free goal setting and progress sheets, and a food diary with an exercise log. If you are self motivated and don't require someone else to set goals for you, or need calorie input and expenditure calculated, this is a good website with lots of useful tools and advice.

Organisations

The British Association for Nutrition and Lifestyle Medicine (BANT)

British Association for Applied Nutrition and Nutritional Therapy
27 Old Gloucester Street, London WC1N 3XX
Telephone: 08706 061284
www.bant.org.uk
BANT is a professional body for registered nutrition practitioners and nutritional therapists. A list of registered practitioners can be found on the BANT website, along with information explaining the differences between dieticians, nutritionists and nutritional therapists.

Complementary and Natural Health Council (CNHC)

https://www.cnhc.org.uk
The CNHC was set up by the government to protect the public. They set the standards for education and qualifications of nutritional therapists and other complementary therapists, and provide a UK register of complementary health practitioners. You can find a registered nutritional therapist on their database.

British Nutrition Foundation

High Holborn House, 52-54 High Holborn. London. WC1V 6RQ
Tel: 0207 4046504
www.nutrition.org.uk
The British Nutrition Foundation is a credible source of nutrition information. It provides reliable information on food, nutrition and healthy eating, as well as topical news items and scientific research.

Books

Dr Atkins' New Diet Revolution
Robert C. Atkins. Vermilion, London (1999)
For an in depth review of ketosis including information from research trials, and a guide to following a ketogenic diet.

Food Doctor Diet Book
Ian Barber. Dorling Kindersley Limited, London (2003)
For lots of healthy eating plans and recipes.

Get into Running
Sara Kirkham. Hodder Headline, London (2010) £9.99
For help beginning or maintaining a running habit, including exercise psychology to help you to stick with it, sample running menus, and running programmes from starting out up to half marathon.

GI How to succeed using a Glycaemic Index diet
Harper Collins. HarperCollins Publishers, Glasgow (2005)
For a 'traffic light' easy reference guide to high, medium and low GI foods.

Lose Weight, Gain Energy, Get Healthy
Sara Kirkham. Hodder Headline, London (2010) £7.99
For healthy eating plans and recipes, a detox programme, a superfood eating plan, and information on how your diet affects your health, energy levels and how you age.

The Fat-Loss Plan: 100 Quick and Easy Recipes with Workouts
Joe Wicks. Bluebird, London.
For recipes and workouts to help weight loss.

The PK Cookbook
Dr. Sarah Myhill and Craig Robinson. Hammersmith Health Books, London.
For an overview of ketosis, recipes and a very simplified, easy way of eating on a ketogenic diet.

Journal articles / references

Antoni R, Johnston KL, Collins AL, Robertson MD. Intermittent v. continuous energy restriction: differential effects on postprandial glucose and lipid metabolism following matched weight loss in overweight/obese participants. *British Journal of Nutrition*, 2018, Volume 119(5):507-516. doi: 10.1017/S0007114517003890.

Barnosky AR, Hoddy KK, Unterman TG, Varady KA. Intermittent fasting vs daily calorie restriction for type 2 diabetes prevention: a review of human findings. *Translational Research – the journal of laboratory and clinical medicine*, 2014, Volume 164:302–311.

Barr SB and Wright JC. Postprandial energy expenditure in whole-food and processed-food meals: implications for daily energy expenditure. *Food and Nutrition Research*, 2010, Volume 2;54. doi: 10.3402/fnr.v54i0.5144.

Bigaard J, Frederiksen K, Tjønneland A, Thomsen BL, Overvad K, Heitmann BL, Sørensen TI. Waist circumference and body composition in relation to all-cause mortality in middle-aged men and women. *International Journal of Obesity*, 2005, Volume 29(7): 778-84.

Björntorp P, Carlgren G, Isaksson B, Krotkiewski M, Larsson B, and Sjöström L. 'Effect of an energy-reduced dietary regimen in relation to adipose tissue cellularity in obese women'. *The American Journal of Clinical Nutrition*, 1975, Vol 28, Issue 5: 445-452. Available at: http://www.ncbi.nlm.nih.gov/sites/entrez

Bray GA and Greenway FL Pharmacological Treatment of the Overweight Patient. *Pharmacological Reviews*, 2007, Vol 59, Issue 2: 151-184. Available at: http://pharmrev.aspetjournals.org/content/59/2/151.long

Dehghan M, Mente A, Zhang X, Swaminathan S, Li W, Mohan V, Iqbal R, Kumar R, Wentzel-Viljoen E, Rosengren A, Amma LI, Avezum A, Chifamba J, Diaz R, Khatib R, Lear S, Lopez-Jaramillo P, Liu X, Gupta R, Mohammadifard N, Gao N, Oguz A, Ramli AS, Seron P, Sun Y, Szuba A, Tsolekile L, Wielgosz A, Yusuf R, Hussein Yusufali A, Teo KK, Rangarajan S, Dagenais G, Bangdiwala SI, Islam S, Anand SS, Yusuf S.; Prospective Urban Rural Epidemiology (PURE) study investigators. ssociations of fats and carbohydrate intake with cardiovascular disease and mortality in 18countries from five continents (PURE): a prospective cohort study. *Lancet*. 2017, Volume 4;390(10107):2050-2062. doi: 10.1016/S0140-6736(17)32252-3.

Gibson AA, Seimon RV, Lee CM, Ayre J, Franklin J, Markovic TP, Caterson ID, Sainsbury A. Do ketogenic diets really suppress appetite? A systematic review and meta-analysis.

Obesity Review, 2015, Volume16(1):64-76. doi: 10.1111/obr.12230.

Hall KD and Guo J. Obesity Energetics: Body Weight Regulation and the Effects of Diet Composition. Gastroenterology 2017, Volume 152(7):1718-1727.e3. doi: 10.1053/j.gastro.2017.01.052.

Harvie MN and Howell T. Could Intermittent Energy Restriction and Intermittent Fasting Reduce Rates of Cancer in Obese, Overweight, and Normal-Weight Subjects? A Summary of Evidence. Advances in Nutrition, 2016, Volume 15;7(4):690-705. doi: 10.3945/an.115.011767.

Kral TV, Roe LS, Rolls BJ. Combined effects of energy density and portion size on energy intake in women. American Journal of Clinical Nutrition, 2004, Vol 79, Issue 6: 962-8. Available at: http://www.ncbi.nlm.nih.gov/pubmed/15159224?itool=EntrezSystem2.PEntrez.Pubmed.Pubmed_ResultsPanel.Pubmed_RVDocSum&ordinalpos=15.

Leaf A and Antonio J The Effects of Overfeeding on Body Composition: The Role of Macronutrient Composition – A Narrative Review. International Journal of Exercise Science, 2017, Volume 10(8): 1275–1296.

Longo VD, Mattson MP. Fasting: molecular mechanisms and clinical applications. Cell Metabolism, 2014, Volume 4;19(2):181-92. doi: 10.1016/j.cmet.2013.12.008.

Maillard F, Pereira B, Boisseau N. Effect of High-Intensity Interval Training on Total, Abdominal and Visceral Fat Mass: A Meta-Analysis. Sports Medicine, 2018, Volume 48(2):269-288. doi: 10.1007/s40279-017-0807-y.

Mumme K and Stonehouse W. Effects of medium-chain triglycerides on weight loss and body composition: a meta-analysis of randomized controlled trials. Journal of the Academy of Nutrition and Dietetics, 2015, Volume 115(2):249-63. doi: 10.1016/j.jand.2014.10.022.

Salans LB, Cushman SW and Weismann RE. Studies of Human Adipose Tissue. Adipose Cell Size and Number in Non-obese and Obese Patients. The Journal of Clinical Investigation, 1973, Volume 52, Issue 4: 929-941. Available at: http://www.ncbi.nlm.nih.gov/pmc/articles/PMC302341/?tool=pubmed.

St-Onge MP and Bosarge A. Weight-loss diet that includes consumption of medium-chain triacylglycerol oil leads to a greater rate of weight and fat mass loss than does olive oil. The American Journal of Clinical Nutrition, 2008, Volume 87(3):621-6.

Thivel D, Masurier J, Baquet G, Timmons BW, Pereira B, Berthoin S, Duclos M, Aucouturier J. High-intensity interval training in overweight and obese children and adolescents: systematic review and meta-analysis. The Journal of Sports Medicine and Physical Fitness, 2018. doi: 10.23736/S0022-4707.18.08075-1.

Westerterp KR. Diet induced thermogenesis. Nutrition and Metabolism, 2004, Volume 1: 5.

Wewege M, van den Berg R, Ward RE, Keech A. *The effects of high-intensity interval training vs. moderate-intensity continuous training on body composition in overweight and obese adults: a systematic review and meta-analysis. Obesity Reviews*, 2017, Volume 18(6):635-646. doi: 10.1111/obr.12532.

Appendix A

A healthy 7 day eating plan for weight loss and weight maintenance

Monday

Breakfast Poached eggs (1-2) on a bed of spinach or with asparagus

Lunch Chicken/turkey or fish and vegetables in a homemade soup

Dinner Baked/grilled salmon/beef/tofu with vegetables in a stir fry

Tuesday

Breakfast CoYo coconut or Greek yoghurt with 1 tablespoon nuts (choose from almonds, pecans, brazils, hazelnuts, walnuts, cashews, chestnuts)

Lunch Fish or meat or mixed pulses with salad: grated carrot, bean sprouts, celery, rocket, tomatoes, cucumber, beetroot and onion

Dinner Seared tuna or beef steak with purple sprouting broccoli, roasted/baked peppers, mushrooms, courgette and red onion

Wednesday

Breakfast Spinach, orange and banana smoothie (see recipe)

Lunch Sardines or turkey with a green salad: rocket, watercress or spinach, olives, pine nuts, grated carrots, beetroot, tomatoes and red onion

Dinner Omelette with red onion/mushrooms/rocket/tomatoes, with side salad

Thursday

Breakfast CoYo coconut or Greek yoghurt with seeds (pumpkin, linseed, sesame, sunflower, fennel)

Lunch Chicken, turkey or vegetable broth

Dinner Feta cheese and spinach soufflé – see recipe

Friday

Breakfast Spinach and cantaloupe melon smoothie

Lunch Tuna or any other fish, or prawns, crab, any other shellfish, with a mixed salad. Lean meat, eggs or pulses can be eaten instead.

Dinner Salmon and avocado salad with celery, mixed green leaves, chicory, cucumber and beetroot

Saturday

Breakfast Egg and banana pancake – see recipe

Lunch Mozzerella and vine tomatoes on a bed of rocket, sprinkle of olive oil

Dinner Courgette or carrot 'spaghetti' made with a Spiralizer with onions, mushrooms, peppers and topped with 10g grated parmesan cheese and/ or a tablespoon of pine nuts

Sunday

Breakfast Smoked mackerel/kippers with a poached egg and field mushroom

Lunch Roast Sunday dinner (exclude or limit Yorkshire pudding, potatoes)

Dinner Chicken or turkey broth

If snacks are necessary between meals, choose from raw vegetables (carrot, cucumber, red/yellow/orange pepper, cucumber, celery sticks, mange tout, asparagus, cherry tomatoes), nuts, pieces of fresh coconut, olives, nut/seed bars (try Nakd bars/Primal pantry or make your own). If you are choosing to extend your overnight fast, breakfast can be missed or eaten later, or lunch eaten as a brunch. Protein foods (meat, fish, seafood, eggs, tofu, beans) should be approximately a palm sized portion; salad and other vegetables can be larger portions.

Drink water throughout the day.

Appendix B

Recipes

Smoothies

If making a smoothie, always include a handful of spinach or kale to reduce the glycaemic index of the meal, slowing down absorption of sugars from fruit. Dark green leaves also provide many essential nutrients. Blend a handful of spinach/kale with a handful of any fruit and add water. Good combinations include:

- Spinach/kale and cantaloupe melon, with enough water to blend
- Spinach/kale and a handful of any one type of mixed berries, and water
- Spinach/kale and half a banana and an orange, and water

Banana and egg pancake (Serves 2)

1 banana
2 eggs
A little coconut or olive oil
Ground almonds (optional)

Blend the banana with the egg to make a batter, then add to a pan to make small pancakes, using oil if required. Brown on each side and serve with a little yoghurt, flaked almonds and berries.

Feta cheese and spinach soufflé (Serves 2)

1 teaspoon olive oil
1 pack of feta cheese (other cheese will do)
1 onion
2 – 3 handfuls of spinach
2 cloves garlic
1 egg, beaten

You can add fresh tomatoes or any other vegetables to this mixture. It will make 2 – 3 ramekins of savoury soufflé which you can eat hot or cold.

Brown chopped onion and garlic with a little oil, then mix together with one egg, and the cheese and spinach. Bake for 40 minutes at 180°C.

Vegetable (superfood) curry (Serves 2 – 4)

1 teaspoon olive oil
1 small tin of chickpeas
1 onion
1 large sweet potato
2 cloves garlic
3 large fresh tomatoes
2 heaped teaspoons turmeric
2 carrots
Handful of fresh coriander
1 small pot fat free Greek yoghurt
2 red chillies, chopped
1 vegetable stock cube made into 300ml
1 head of broccoli

Heat the oil, cooking the garlic and onion until soft. Add a teaspoon of finely chopped coriander, turmeric and chillies. Stir and cook for 2 minutes. Add carrots, sweet potato and tomatoes. Add the liquid stock and chick peas, bring to the boil and then simmer for approximately 20 minutes. Meanwhile, blanch the broccoli and add once the curry is cooked. Remove from the heat; allow to cool slightly before adding the yoghurt. Sprinkle a generous helping of fresh coriander on top and serve with brown rice (60g per person, uncooked weight).

Mediterranean Salad

1 large avocado
3 large fresh tomatoes (or drained sun-dried)
1 ball mozzarella
2 carrots
Olive oil
2 large handfuls of rocker
Cucumber
2 tablespoons of pine nuts
1 handful of asparagus

Griddle the asparagus. Meanwhile, put together the salad by mixing rocket, tomatoes, torn mozzarella, chunks of cucumber, olives and avocado in a bowl with a drizzle of olive oil. Place a serving on each plate and place the asparagus on top, and drizzle with a little balsamic vinegar.

Savoy cabbage stir fry (Serves 2)

One onion
Two cloves of garlic
One Savoy cabbage
Mushrooms, peppers, peas, sweet corn or mange tout as desired
Baked beans or tinned tomatoes for the sauce
A little olive oil or coconut oil

Heat a little olive oil in a pan. Add a chopped onion and one or two cloves of sliced garlic. Any herbs or spices can also be added at this time (such as chopped chili). Cut the Spring cabbage into thin strips and add this to the pan. Once the onion and cabbage are slightly browned, add the other vegetables such as mushrooms, frozen peas, sweet corn or baby corn, mange tout and strips of fresh or frozen peppers. A portion of tofu, chicken or turkey can be added at this stage too, and half a tin of baked beans or tinned tomatoes can be used to create a sauce – just add to the mix and stir until heated through.

Stuffed vegetables (Serves 2)

2 large peppers, raw, with tops cut off
2 potatoes
1 onion, chopped
2 cloves of garlic, chopped
100g fresh spinach
1 handful each of mushrooms, fresh or frozen sweet corn and peas
1 dessertspoon of mixed seeds
1 teaspoon of olive oil

Bake the potatoes until cooked. Meanwhile, heat a little oil and lightly stir fry the garlic, mushroom and onion. Add the peas and sweet corn and heat through, adding the spinach. Stir until wilted and remove from the heat. Cut off the top of the potatoes, scoop out the mash into the stir fry and mix. Once thoroughly mixed, stuff the peppers and potatoes with the mixture of stir-fried onions, garlic, mushrooms, peas, spinach, sweet corn, and mixed seeds and bake for 35 minutes at 180°C/gas mark 4. Serve with a large green salad.

Seared tuna/sword fish/marlin steak with stir fry vegetables (Serves 2)

1 onion
1 handful of mushrooms
2 cloves of garlic
1 cupful of mixed sweet corn and peas
1 fresh pepper
1 teaspoon sesame seeds
2 tuna steaks
Olive oil

Chop the mushrooms, garlic and onions and add to a teaspoon of heated olive oil in a pan. Once browned, add the chopped peppers, sweet corn and peas, and cook through. Add the seeds and heat for a further few minutes until just browned. Meanwhile, sear the tuna steak in a non-stick pan. You could rub chopped chilli and garlic onto the fish beforehand if you wish. Serve!

Chili bean casserole (Serves 2 – 4)

Any type of beans/lentils, soaked
1 onion, chopped
2 cloves of garlic, chopped
1-2 chilies, chopped
1 tin of tomatoes
75g organic brown rice per person
Cupful of fresh tomatoes
Olive oil
Mushrooms
Carrots, diced
Frozen peas and sweet corn
Fresh/frozen peppers

Soak a selection of beans overnight or choose beans/lentils that require no soaking. If you want a lower carbohydrate chilli, simply add only a small amount (1 small tin or a handful) of beans/lentils, or avoid completely. Whilst boiling the beans/lentils, brown garlic and onion in a little olive oil then add the fresh chilis. Add the carrots, mushrooms and other vegetables to the dish with the tinned tomatoes. Simmer for one hour or as required, adding the beans half way through. Fresh tomatoes may be added if desired, along with any other vegetables, lentils and other pulses not requiring pre-soaking. Serve with brown rice (50g dry weight per person) or a small baked potato.